Rosemary Gladstar's
Herbal
Remedies *for*
CHILDREN'S
HEALTH

STOREY
BOOKS

Dedication

To my first grandchild, Andrew Colvard: may this tradition live on in your veins. May we take care of the plants in such a way that they remain in sweet abundance for your generation and future ones, so that you may walk upon the Earth 50 or 100 years from now, hand in hand with your grandson, showing him the good medicines of the Earth.

The mission of Storey Communications is to serve our customers by publishing practical information that encourages personal independence in harmony with the environment.

This publication is intended to provide educational information for the reader on the covered subject. It is not intended to take the place of personalized medical counseling, diagnosis, and treatment from a trained health professional.

Edited by Deborah Balmuth and Robin Catalano
Cover design by Carol Jessop, Black Trout Design, and Meredith Maker
Back cover photograph by A. Blake Gardner
Cover and interior illustrations by Laura Tedeschi
Text design by Carol Jessop, Black Trout Design
Text production by Susan B. Bernier
Indexed by Nan Badgett, Word•a•bil•i•ty

Printed in Canada by Webcom Limited
10 9 8 7 6 5 4 3 2

Library of Congress Cataloging-in-Publication Data

Gladstar, Rosemary
   [Herbal remedies for children's health]
   Rosemary Gladstar's herbal remedies for children's health / Rosemary Gladstar.
      p.   cm.
   Includes bibliographical references and index.
   ISBN 1-58017-153-2 (pbk. : alk. paper)
   1. Herbs — Therapeutic use. 2. Children — Diseases — Alternative treatment.
3. Materia medica, Vegetable. 4. Children — Health and hygiene. 5. Naturopathy. I. Title
RM666.H33G533   1999
615'.321'083 — dc21   99-10045
                                                          CIP

CONTENTS

Preface

As I finish the last pages of this book, I am getting ready for my sister-in-law and her two beautiful daughters, Samantha, 10, and Lindsey, 6, to come for an overnight visit. They are also bringing their friend, Marissa, who is 11, and already filled with the love of plants. This will be a special "herb visit" with the girls and "Aunt Rosie." I've been planning for the last few days the things I wish to do with them. There's so much that's green and beautiful. We'll make my famous herbal face cream and maybe do herbal steams and facials. I've got great little containers for handmade lip balms that we'll color red with the root of alkanet, a flower I grow in my garden.

It's autumn and the golden leaves of New England have woven a rich tapestry upon the forest floor. Though it's raining out, we'll undoubtedly take a long walk through the golden forest, drinking in the colors once again before the long winter sets in, seeing if there's still a plant here and there to identify and harvest. I'm thinking, too, of stories that will be fun to tell by the campfire tonight. We're going to camp out in the yurt, a round tent structure with a woodstove that will keep us warm and snug, even though the weather is already beginning to turn in the mountains of Vermont.

It is times like these that I am reminded most of my own childhood and my early encouters with plants. I am forever thankful for the lessons my grandmother taught me as a child in her gardens. No matter how little you think you may know about the plants — or how much — that knowledge is a gift to pass on. What we learn to love as children, we will love and respect as adults.

chapter one

The Benefits of an Herbal Approach for Children

A long time ago, when I was just a child, my grandmother took me into her gardens and introduced me to her weeds. When we walked in the scented oak forest, she would rub my skin with fresh bay leaves, assuring me it would prevent poison oak and would keep the insects from swarming over us. When I fell in the nettle patches, she soothed the painful welts with the fresh juice of that plant.

She showed me how to knit with chicken feathers and taught me special games to play with the shiny, smooth bones she kept on the mantle. Her teachings were without fuss. Strong and powerful, like her, her words sank deep and took root in this young child's heart. That magic my grandmother taught me in the garden of my childhood stayed with me throughout my life, and I have continued the journey into the green.

I've studied the healing power of herbs with many gifted teachers, traveled to many herbally rich areas, come to know a great many more plants, and studied the science as well as the art of herbal healing. Still, the things I learned as a child with my grandmother have remained some of the most powerful teachings of my life. It is what my grandmother taught me in her simple, strong wisdom that I seek to pass on to you and your children.

Herbalism instills in a person a deep appreciation for the Mother Earth and knowledge of natural healing and well-being. Teach children early this love of the Earth, the respect of plants and nature. All children benefit from a close association with nature and from the use of herbs and the ancient tradition of herbalism. What one learns to know and love as a child is often what is treasured most as an adult.

Herbs provide tremendous benefits for children's health. Most of the simple woes of childhood respond quickly to herbal therapies. Cuts, burns, bee stings, colds, and runny noses become opportunities for you and your children to see how effectively herbal remedies work. Even the more tenacious childhood illnesses such as chicken pox and measles, flus, fevers, and allergies respond to the healing power of herbs. When it's necessary to resort to allo-pathic medication, herbs provide a wonderful complement, helping to support the child's system while the medication does its work. A simple knowledge of herbs and a well-stocked herbal pantry can lessen the trials of childhood illnesses considerably.

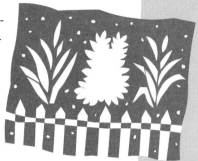

Understanding Plants' Healing Powers

For ages, long before we had computers, technology, libraries, or even herb books, people knew and understood the healing power of herbs. I am convinced that this knowing came from an intrinsic sense of the plant. It was not simply a trial-and-error process, as we often claim, that people learned about the plant spirit and medicine.

Although trial and error played a part in our understanding, most of what we know about plant medicines came through and from the plants themselves.

Children's Connections with the Plant Spirits

Mary, a practicing herbalist who lives in Tahoe, California, had a beautiful herb garden. Her youngest daughter, Amber, loved being in the garden. When Amber was three years old, she became enthralled by the fairies and flower spirits that lived in the garden. She convinced her mom to make miniature garden settings for the fairies, to set up tea parties with tiny greeting cards and little flower-covered archways.

LISTENING TO NATURE

Plants have an innate way of communicating with people, and I believe that most anybody can learn to listen to the plants. However, there are certain people who lend an ear more readily to the songs, or voices, of the plants. These people are generally termed keepers of the green, green witches, herbalists, healers, or other, more derogatory titles, depending on which day and age you live in.

Mary delighted in this summer pastime and her daughter's sense of enchantment. But then, quite suddenly, Amber couldn't sleep at night. Around midnight, she'd come to her parents' doorway and ask to sleep with them. "The fairies won't leave me alone," she'd tell them, "they are stringing lights all over my room and waking me with their singing." And father and mother, half asleep, would let their little daughter crawl under the covers with them.

One night, they decided enough was enough and Amber must go back to her own room to sleep. But when they got to the door, Mary tells me in a voice still hushed after these many years, they heard ringing and singing. And when they opened the door, there were miniature lights dancing about the room.

I love this story because there are still many children who hear the songs of the plants. They talk to the plants and the plants "talk" back. They seem to know what to pick to put on their "owies." And they'd much rather be out in the garden than sitting mindlessly in front of the TV.

Nurturing Herbal Wisdom in Today's World

In native cultures around the world, children who had a special gift with the plants were recognized early. Often tutored by their grandparents or the elders of the village, their training began in childhood. It continued long into adulthood and generally involved a lengthy, rigorous apprenticeship with the local herbalist, community healer, or shaman. These people then became the healers of their communities, and so the tradition was carried on down through the ages.

Still today, we have those children who are "plant sensitives," who seem to carry a gene of "green blood" in them. You recognize them at family gatherings, on the playground, in school. Girls and boys — gender isn't relevant — are often found looking at the flowers, lost in play for hours in the gardens, enchanted by the pollen-covered insects and butterflies lazing on the launching pads of freshly opened blossoms. They take special delight in resting their heads on the moss-covered rocks. They play games with the flowers and woodland plants and seem to have a special rapport with all of nature. Watch for those children. In the old days, they were the "keepers of the green," and were recognized as future wise ones and healers.

Though herbology is generally recognized and honored as our oldest system of healing, much of the art of herbalism is at risk today. In teaching our children how to use herbs as a way of life and instilling in them a respect for this ancient tradition, we not only care for our children's tender bodies, but help to pass along the seeds of a tradition that is as old as human life itself.

Practicing Herbal Medicine

In traditional cultures, the herb pickers or gatherers were trained to ask permission from the plant itself before harvesting it for medicine. This was considered not only essential in retaining the healing power of the plant, but also respectful, a simple courtesy. If one picked the plant without prayer or thanksgiving, then the medicine of the plant stayed in the earth. Now that makes sense, doesn't it? It also makes sense when trying to determine a remedy or an appropriate treatment, that one considers asking the plant directly — not in place of adequate research and study, but in addition to it. The plants are here to help us, and asking for their help is one step in understanding them.

MAYAN PRAYER FOR PICKING PLANTS

In the name of God the Father, God the Son, and God the Holy Spirit, I am the one searching for the plants to heal the people. I give thanks to the spirit of this plant, and I have faith with all my heart that this plant will heal the sickness of [person's name].

For instance, when I'm harvesting plants for medicine, I ask permission first, from the plant, to use its healing power. And sometimes when I'm trying to find an appropriate remedy or combination of herbs, I ask the plants directly. It's a "feeling" or sensing I get about which plant is right. I don't think this is a special gift. I think it's something many people have, but they forget to use it. As you become more familiar working with plants and using herbal remedies, you might wish to try this technique.

Using Herbs for Children's Health Care

Not only do herbs serve as wonderful teachers for our children, they also provide an effective, gentle system of healing for them. Children's bodies are sensitive and respond naturally and quickly to the healing energy of herbs. I believe this is because there is an inborn wisdom that is still strongly connected; the "umbilical cord" is still deeply entwined with the body of the Earth Mother and the many gifts that flow like a life-giving stream from her core. Administered wisely, herbs do not upset the delicate ecological balance of children's small bodies as does much of modern medicine, but rather work in harmony with the young child's system.

When to Use Herbs

Herbs can be used with confidence for simple ailments such as colds, colic, and teething, as well as the many common childhood illnesses that children often contract. Herbs can also be used as supplements to our modern system of allopathic medicine when dealing with more complicated health problems. Contrary to popular opinion, herbs and orthodox medicine are not at odds, but are two systems of healing that can complement one another. Consult your physician or holistic health care provider for guidelines on using allopathic drugs and herbal remedies in combination.

When to Seek Medical Help

Though herbs are often helpful, no one system of medicine works for all illnesses, or in all situations. Allopathic medicine is an excellent emergency- or crisis-oriented system; in fact, it is the best system for life-threatening situations. It is important to know when to seek medical help for your child. Be sure to establish a relationship with a pediatrician, preferably one who is holistically minded, while your child is well.

Seek medical help if the child:

- Is not responding to the herbal treatments you are using.
- Shows signs of serious illness. Some examples are fever greater than 102°F, low-grade persistent fever, hemorrhaging, delirium, unconsciousness, and severe abdominal pain.
- Is lethargic and weak, unresponsive, or difficult to awaken.
- Complains of stiff neck and headache and is unable to touch his or her chin to the chest. In babies, the fontanel (soft spot on top of the head) may bulge. These are possible early signs of meningitis, and require immediate medical assistance.
- Contracts recurring ear infections.
- Shows any signs of choking on a foreign object; these include difficulty breathing, sucking in breath, and turning blue.
- Becomes dehydrated. Warning signs are dry lips and inside of mouth, and absence of urination in 6 hours.
- Has bee stings or insect bites that cause allergic reactions and shock. Extreme anxiety, difficulty breathing, and other unusual responses can be warning signs.
- Has red streaks on the skin emanating from the point of infection; this could indicate blood poisoning.
- Exhibits burned areas that cover twice the size of the child's hand or are infected. Aso look for signs of shock and third-degree burns.

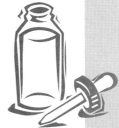

Getting Perspective on the Safety of Herbs

Herbs are among the safest medications available on Earth. This does not mean that there are not toxic plants or herbal remedies that can cause side effects or harmful reactions. But the herbs we use today have been used for centuries by people around the world. Until recently, studies of herbs were conducted on people, not laboratory animals, so we have a pretty good idea of how herbs work on the human body and the reactions they cause.

Herbs that have toxic side effects have been noted and well documented, and most of these herbs, wisely, are not available for sale in this country. Occasionally, an herb will stimulate an idiosyncratic reaction in an individual. This doesn't make the herb toxic, just a poor choice for that particular individual. Strawberries, a perfectly delicious fruit, are sweet nectar to some and a noxious substance to others.

Using Herbs Wisely

There are many reports surfacing these days about the toxicity of herbs. Even perfectly benign substances such as chamomile and peppermint are winding up on the "black list." I think the reason for this is not that more people are using herbs (as is often suggested), but that people are using herbs in ways that allow greater amounts of and more concentrated dosages. In the past, herbs were most often taken as teas and syrups, in baths and salves, and in tinctures and extracts. Herbal capsules that allow for greater numbers of dosages and standardized preparations that are far beyond the normal concentrations found in nature have not been available until recently.

With not centuries but millennia of experience behind the use of medicinal herbs, you can be assured of the safety of both you and your child. But you must follow the appropriate dosages outlined in this book, use only those herbs that have a record of safety, and respond quickly by discontinuing an herb if you suspect it to be the cause of an idiosyncratic response.

chapter two

The Children's Herbal Medicine Chest

Contrary to what you may have heard or read, my experience has been that almost any herb that is safe for an adult is safe for a child as long as the size and weight of the child are accounted for and the dosage is adjusted accordingly. However, some herbs are far better suited to the more sensitive constitutions of children and should always be considered first. People often express concern about using strong medicinal herbs such as goldenseal, valerian, or St.-John's-wort for children, but I've found them to be extremely useful and effective. However, use them in small amounts for short periods of time only, and use them in conjunction, or formulated with, the milder herbs listed in this book.

Safety Precautions

Any herb, even the safest and most researched of herbs, can affect different people differently. Much in the same way that some people get horrendous allergic reactions to strawberries, milk, and plant pollen, some people are adversely affected by even the most benevolent of herbs. Though it is a rare and unusual occurrence, whenever such a reaction is reported it makes national headlines. Were drug reactions reported with the same fervor, we'd have a national headline on aspirin and Zoloft every day. However rare these reactions to herbs may be, it is always wise to be cautious when using an herb for the first time.

Do Small-Dose Tests

Use the herb in small amounts at first, to see how it works for you and your child. A good safety measure is a patch test. Make an herb tea, then "paint" a small amount onto the skin of the inner arm. Wait 24 hours; if you do notice any adverse reactions — skin rash, itchy eyes, throat swelling, itchiness — discontinue use immediately. If the child does not experience an adverse reaction, you may administer a very small amount internally. Discontinue immediately if any signs of allergic reaction appear. You may wish to try the herb again, prepared in the same manner and administered in the same amount, after a few days. If the child experiences discomfort again, then I would attribute the effects to the herb or herbal formula and look for another, more compatible herb.

Buying Quality Herbs

When using herbs, it is important that you insist on high quality organically grown herbs. Though these herbs may cost a few cents more, they are far better for our children and our planet. Have at least two ounces of the herbs you plan to use on hand at all times. Store them properly so they have a long active shelf life. And don't use herbs that are endangered or at risk (see page 73), whether from this country or elsewhere.

Store in Childproof Containers

Herbs retain their properties best if stored in airtight glass jars, out of direct light, in a cool area. If you have small children in your household, store herbs in glass bottles with tight-fitting lids. Be sure to label the jars, for it becomes an impossible task to remember what's what in those little glass bottles. Store medicinal preparations — herbs as well as homeopathic or allopathic medications — out of reach of children. One of the problems with many medicinal preparations, including herbal remedies, is that they are made to taste appealing. Thankfully, most of your herbal remedies won't be harmful if used in larger amounts than intended. Still, out of reach and in well-sealed containers is a good general rule.

Herbs and Their Uses

The herbs listed in this chapter are the ones I recommend you start with and use most often for children's health and healing. These herbs have a gentle and sure action with no residual buildup or side effects in the body. These "gentle" herbs can be very strong, but they act in a softer, less abrasive manner than lobelia, chaparral, or cascara. If I must use stronger medicinals, I *always* formulate them with these gentler, "child-friendly" herbs.

Anise (Pimpinella anisum)

Parts used: primarily seeds, but leaves are useful

Benefits: Anise is a carminative (gas-expelling), warming digestive aid. It has a tasty licorice-like flavor that most children enjoy.

Suggested uses: Use as a tea for colic and other digestive problems. Because of its sweet flavor, anise is often blended with less tasty herbs.

Astragalus (Astragalus membranaceus)

Parts used: root

Benefits: Adaptogenic (resistance-building) and toning, astragalus sometimes is called the young person's ginseng. While echinacea supports the immune system's first line of defense, astragalus strengthens the deep immune system by helping rebuild the bone marrow reserve that regenerates the body's protective shield.

Suggested uses: Astragalus is best used in tea for long-term illness, low energy, and to support and build immunity. The root looks exactly like the tongue depressors doctors use, and can be a bit tricky to work with. Place a whole or chopped root or two in a pot of soup or water and simmer for several hours. Astragalus also can be served in capsules. Children enjoy chewing on the root like they do licorice sticks.

HERBAL HISTORY

Our Puritan forefathers (and mothers!) used to mix carminitive (digestive-aiding) seeds such as anise, dill, fennel, and carway together. They would carry the mixture in little containers to the long church services that the children were forced to sit through. They would chew on these "meetin' seeds" to calm their stomachs, but I'm not sure it calmed their restless spirits.

Borage *(Borago officinalis)*

Parts used: flowers, leaves

Benefits: A traditional plant used for anxiety and stress, borage is especially useful when the spirits need lifting. Even little children get the blues, and this lovely blue-flowered plant can be quite helpful.

Suggested uses: This plant loses much of its medicinal qualities when dried, so use it fresh whenever possible. Make a flower essence from borage (see the many reference books available), or drink a tea made with the flowers and leaves. Drunk throughout the day, borage will help allay depression.

Catnip *(Nepeta cataria)*

Parts used: leaves, flowers

Benefits: This versatile plant is a garden mint that grows easily both in and out of the garden. While it sends cats into spasms of pleasure, it is an excellent calming herb used for all manner of stress. It is particulary benefical for lowering fevers and for the pain of teething. It is also a restorative digestive aid used for indigestion, diarrhea, and colic.

Suggested uses: Serve as a tea throughout the day to alleviate teething pain. Catnip is quite bitter tasting, so combine it with pleasant tasting herbs such as oats and lemon balm. Give a couple drops of the tincture before meals to serve as a digestive aid. A few drops of the tincture before bedtime will help calm a fussy child. This is an excellent herb to help reduce fevers; use both as a tincture and an enema for this purpose.

Chamomile (Martricaria recutita, Anthemis nobilis, and related species)

Parts used: primarily flowers, but leaves are useful

Benefits: This little plant is a healing wonder. It has rich amounts of essential oil in its flower tops that act as a powerful anti-inflammatory agent. The flowers make a wonderfully soothing tea that is good for the nervous system. It also promotes digestion. Chamomile is one of the best herbs for colicky babies.

Suggested uses: Chamomile tea sweetened with honey can be served throughout the day to calm a stressed or nervous child. A massage oil made from chamomile essential oil can be used for similar calming effects, and to soothe sore, achy muscles. A few drops of this tincture will aid digestion; administer before feeding time. Chamomile is frequently added to a baby's bath for a marvelous, soothing wash. This is one of the best all-around children's herbs.

Corn Silk (Zea Mays)

Parts used: golden — not brown — silk of organically grown corn

Benefits: The flower pistils from maize have long been used as a urinary tonic. Corn silk acts as an antiseptic, diruetic, and demulcent on the urinary system, stimulating and cleaning urinary passages while soothing any urinary inflammation.

Suggested uses: One of the most effective herbs for bed-wetting, corn silk can be taken as a tincture at night to help prevent the problem. Use as a tea during the day, ceasing 3 to 4 hours before bedtime, to strenghten the urinary system. *Note:* Other treatments — such as counseling, kegel exercises, and allergy testing — may have to be used in conjunction with the corn silk for the treatment to be effective.

Dill (Anethum graveolens)

Parts used: primarily seeds, but leaves are useful
Benefits: Like anise, dill is a good digestive aid, and has an even greater reputation for expelling gas.
Suggested uses: Dill is used directly in food, ground up and placed in capsules, and brewed in teas for colic- and gas-relieving properties.

Echinacea (Echinacea angustifolia, E. purpurea, and related species)

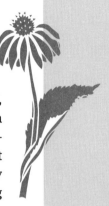

Parts used: roots, leaves, flowers
Benefits: The best immuno-enhancing herb that we know of, and one of the most important herbs of our times, echinacea is beautiful, hearty, and has no known side effects or residual buildup. The *purpurea* species grows easily in most climates and can be planted and tended by children. It is easy to make medicine from echinacea, which works by increasing macrophage T-cell activity, thereby increasing the body's protective shield or first line of defense. Though potent, it is 100% safe for use in children.
Caution: There are several types of echinacea available. Because of the huge demand, echinacea is being poached mercilessly from its wild habitats; avoid wild-harvested varieties. I recommend *E. purpurea* because it is easily grown in the garden and is just as effective as the wild varieties.
Suggested uses: At the first sign of a cold or flu, use echinacea in tea or tincture form to boost immunity. Take it in frequent, small doses. Useful as a tea or tincture for children's bronchial infections. A spray can be made to soothe sore throats. For sore gums and mouth inflammation, make a mouthwash from the root and flavor with peppermint or spearmint essential oil.

Fennel *(Foeniculum vulgare)*

Parts used: primarily seeds, but also leaves and flowers

Benefits: A well-known carminative and digesitive aid, this tall, graceful plant has been used — from the time of the early Greek physicians — to increase and enrich the milk flow in nursing mothers. It is also an antacid that both neutralizes excess acids in the stomach and intestines and clears uric acid from the joints. More generally, it stimulates digestion, regulates appetite, and relieves flatulence.

Suggested uses: A wonderfully tasty fennel tea is used for treating colic, improving digestion, and expelling gas from the system. Use a wash of warm fennel tea for conjunctivitis and other eye inflammations. Nursing mothers can drink two to four cups daily to increase and enrich their flow of milk. Because of its delightful licorice-like flavor, it's a great flavoring agent for less tasty herbs.

Fenugreek *(Trigonella foenum-graecum)*

Parts used: seeds

Benefits: One of the earliest medicines mentioned in the recorded annals of herbalism, fenugreek seeds are rich in oil and mucilage. They are exceptionally nourishing and are used to treat debilitating and wasting disorders. They are soothing to irritated membranes in the throat and stomach. The seeds help regulate blood sugar levels and improve glucose tolerance. Fenugreek is also good for children and adults who have trouble gaining weight.

Suggested uses: Because of its bitter flavor, fenugreek will definitely have to be formulated with other herbs to make it palatable. Combine fenugreek seeds with other herbs to create a wash for sore, irritated throats and digestive tracts. Nursing mothers can take fenugreek tea to help enrich their flow of milk.

Hibiscus (Hibiscus sabdariffa and related species)

Parts used: flowers
Benefits: High in vitamin C and bioflavonoids, hibiscus has slightly astringent properties. It is useful for treating mild colds, flus, bruising, and swelling.
Suggested uses: The large tropical hibiscus flowers make a beautiful ruby red tea, and children adore it. The flavor is somewhat tart with a sweet aftertaste. Children often prefer to have it sweetened even more, and I'll frequently mix hibiscus with stevia or other sweet herbs to enhance the flavor.

Lemon Balm (Melissa officinalis)

Parts used: leaves
Benefits: Calming, antiviral, and antiseptic, this beautifully fragrant member of the mint family is one of nature's best nervine herbs. It is used as a mild sedative.
Suggested uses: Lemon balm makes a delicious tea and can be served with lemon and honey throughout the day to alleviate stress and anxiety. For a delicious nervine tonic, blend equal amounts of lemon balm, oats, and chamomile. Fresh lemon balm is preferred for medicinal preparations.

Licorice (Glycyrrhiza glabra)

Parts used: root
Benefits: The effective yet delicious qualities of this herb help make it one of the most important herbal remedies for children. It is used for a multitude of ailments including bronchial congestion, sore throat, coughs, and inflammation of the digestive tract (such as ulcers or nonspecific sores).
Caution: Though most children don't suffer from these ailments, licorice should not be used in children who have hypertension or kidney/bladder problems, or those youngsters on steroid therapy.
Suggested uses: Licorice is very sweet and often must be blended with other herbs to be palatable. Use in syrups, teas, and washes. Children enjoy chewing on licorice sticks.

Marsh Mallow (Althaea officinalis)

Parts used: primarily roots, but leaves and flowers are useful
Benefits: This soothing, mucilaginous herb can be used like slippery elm, but is much more readily available and is easy to grow in most garden settings.
Suggested uses: Serve as a tea for sore throats, diarrhea, constipation, and bronchial inflammation. Mix into a paste with water to soothe irritated skin. Marsh mallow can also be used in the bath along with oatmeal for a soothing wash.

Nettle (Urtica dioica)

Parts used: fresh leaves, young tops
Benefits: High in vitamins and minerals, especially iron and calcium, nettle is an excellent remedy for allergies and hay fever. It's useful for alleviating growing pains in young children.
Suggested uses: Nettle is pleasant tasting, and is often steamed and served as a mineral-rich addition to meals. It can be used to replace spinach in any recipe, but always must be well-steamed; it will "sting" you if undercooked! I often serve this herb on toast, or in omelettes, soups, and spinach-nettle pies. A delicious nettle tea can be served several times a day to prevent allergic attacks. Freeze-dried nettle capsules have the best reputation for treating allergies and hay fever, but I often combine the capsules with tea.

ROASTING MARSH MALLOW AT THE CAMPFIRE?

Who would believe that the mucilangeous root of this common herb was the original marsh mallow, the one that kids love to roast over an open fire? Our pioneer parents cooked the root with honey or sugar and formed it into soft balls on which their children could suck to remedy a sore throat.

Oats *(Avena sativa)*

Parts used: The green milky tops of the oat are preferred, but stems can also be used. Best used partially green, before the plant has turned golden.

Benefits: One of the best nutritive tonics for the nervous system, this herb is recommended for nervous exhaustion, stress, and irritation. It is rich in mucilaginous properties, which makes it particulary helpful for damage to the myelin sheath. Oats are high in silica and calcium.

Suggested uses: Both the milky green tops and stalks of oats make a delicious tea — one of the best, I think. Make it strong and mix with fruit juice. Use for children who are nervous, hyperactive, or stressed. Because of its rich mucilaginous content, it makes a wonderfully soothing bath for skin irritations.

Peppermint *(Mentha x piperita)*

Parts used: leaves, flowers

Benefits: Peppermint often has been called "a blast of pure green energy." It's not that there aren't stronger stimulants, but few make you feel as renewed and refreshed as peppermint. Commonly used as a digestive aid, peppermint is effective for easing nausea and stomach cramps, and in clearing the mouth of foul tastes.

Suggested uses: Use for children when they have sluggish digestion and need a burst of "green energy." Peppermint can be made into a tea, tincture (diluted), and mouthwash. Peppermint is most refreshing when just grazed from the garden. I like to introduce children to this safe and tasty plant. Like spearmint, peppermint is a common ingredient in toothpaste and tooth powders.

Red Clover (Trifolium pratense)

Parts used: flowering top, leaves

Benefits: One of the best respiratory tonics, red clover is used for children who have chronic chest complaints such as coughs, colds, and bronchitis. Red clover is rich in minerals, most notably calcium, nitrogen, and iron. It is used for all skin conditions, as it is an excellent detoxifier or blood purifier.

Caution: Do not use consistently for hemophiliacs or people with "thin" blood, as the herb can exacerbate this condition.

Suggested uses: Red clover makes a delicious tea. Blend with other herbs such as mullein for persistent respiratory problems. In addition, you can use the tea for building blood and improving the skin. The tea or tincture can be used when there are growths on the body such as cysts, tumors, and fibroids.

Red Raspberry (Rubus idaeus)

Parts used: leaf, young shoots, fruits

Benefits: Raspberry was first cited in Chinese herbal writings dating back to A.D. 550. It has been used as a uterine tonic and nutritive supplement ever since. Raspberry leaves are rich in vitamins and minerals, particulary calcium and iron.

Suggested uses: As a tea or tincture, raspberry leaf is valuable for diarrhea and dysentery. It helps reduce excessive menstruation and is a superior tonic for use during pregnancy and childbirth. Because of it's astringent properties, raspberry is a good mouthwash for sore or infected gums.

Rose Hips (Rosa canina and related species)

Parts used: primarily seeds, but also leaves and flowers

Benefits: Rose hips contain more vitamin C than almost any other herb, many times the amount found in citrus fruit. Vitamin C is a noted anitoxidant with disease-fighting capabilities. The leaves are astringent and toning. The flowers are used in love potions and flower essences.

Suggested uses: Make fresh rose hips into a vitamin-rich syrup or jam. (Dried seedless rose hips also make a delicious jam. Soak overnight in just enough fresh apple juice to cover. The next day the jam is ready to eat. You also can add cinnamon and other spices.

Rose hips also are used in a delicious, mild-flavored tea.

Slippery Elm (Ulmus fulva, U. rubra)

Parts used: inner bark
Benefits: Slippery elm is one of the most beloved herbs for children. This plant is used for soothing any and all inflammations, internal or external. It is particulary valuable for burns, sore throats, and digestive problems including diarrhea and constipation. A highly nourishing food, it was at one time sold as a medicinal flour and used in cooking
Caution: Many trees have been destroyed by Dutch elm disease. Use slippery elm sparingly, and buy only farm-grown or ethically harvested bark from limbs of fallen trees.
Suggested uses: In a blender, mix 1 tablespoon slippery elm, 1 teaspoon cinnammon, 1 cup warm water, and 1 tablespoon honey. Blend well. Use as a cough medicine. To make a tea, simmer 1 teaspoon of slippery elm in 1 cup hot water. The rather sweet flavor of this herb combines well with others such as licorice, fennel, and cinammon.

SLIPPERY ELM LOZENGES

The discomfort of burns in the mouth can be eased with Slippery Elm Lozenges.

To make the lozenges, mix 1 tablespoon finely ground slippery elm powder with a teaspoon of honey and just enough water to make a paste. Roll into a ball, adding more herb, if needed, to thicken. If the burn is serious, a *tiny* drop of peppermint oil can be added. Suck on the lozenge, using as many as needed until the pain is gone.

Spearmint *(Mentha spicata)*

Parts used: leaves, flowers
Benefits: Cooling, refreshing, and uplifting, spearmint is, with the possible exception of peppermint, the most popular of all mints. It has a crisp, stimulating flavor that can be used to improve the flavors of less tasty herbs.
Suggested uses: Use spearmint to "sweeten" the stomach and breath after sickness, especially vomiting. Add a drop of the essential oil to water or make a cup of fresh tea and rinse the mouth out several times. This herb can be added to uplifting, refreshing tea blends. Spearmint is a nice addition to honey and other foods for a quick pick-me-up.

Stevia *(Stevia rebaudiana)*

Parts used: leaves
Benefits: Called the sweet herb, stevia is sweeter than sugar but much better for you. It has no calories and doesn't promote tooth decay. Stevia is used for pancreatic imbalances and high blood sugar levels. It is a type of sugar that diabetics can tolerate.
Suggested uses: Because of its intense sweetness, it is primarily used to enhance the flavor of other herbs. The only problem is that it is far too sweet. Go lightly.

Wild Cherry *(Prunus serotina)*

Parts used: inner bark
Benefits: This expectorant herb is one of the best for calming most types of coughs. It is one of the few herbs still included in the United States Pharmacopeia's annual drug reference and it is still found in some commerical cough remedies.
Caution: In order not to harm the beautiful trees, I generally collect bark from fallen limbs after a storm.
Suggested uses: A favorite in teas, syrups, and tinctures for coughs and colds, it is also improves digestion and promotes healthy bowel function.

chapter three

Basic Herbal Preparations

Once in a while you'll find that unusual child who will eat every herb you give him or her, no matter how bitter or unpleasant tasting. Both my son and grandson were like that, eager to consume whatever formula they were given.

Andrew, my grandson, seemed to thrive on the flavor of bitter herbs. Whenever he had respiratory problems we would give him a goldenseal formula. Strongly diluted yet still bitterly potent, we'd put the formula in a one-ounce dropper bottle. Andrew would run around with his herbal remedy in hand, drinking it like it was apple juice or something as pleasant.

But most often, one will have the opportunity — or challenge depending how you choose to embrace it — to be creative and innovative when designing herbal preparations for children. The flavors of medicinal herbs are unfamiliar, sometimes bitter, pungent, or sour, and children are often unwilling to try them. Sometimes, just because of the discomfort of being ill, they refuse to eat even their favorite foods. Since consistency, when treating both adults and children, is the key to any herb's effectiveness, it is important to develop preparations and recipes that are pleasant and easy to take.

Determining Dosage

There are several different techniques used to determine the proper dosage for children. Like parents who have grown accustomed to the needs of their children, most herbalists rely on years of experience and intuition. When recommending herbs for small children, I base my suggestions on the size of the child, general constitution, the nature of the illness, and the herbs being used. Then I pray and let the spirit of the herbs guide me. This, of course, is balanced with a thorough understanding of the herbs I am using, plus many years of experience.

If you are just beginning your herbal work or if you are using herbs you are unfamiliar with, then you will need to use the following charts. They provide sound guidelines for prescribing the proper amount of herbs for children. But use the charts just as guidelines; it is equally important to consider the weight and overall health of the child. Also consider the nature of the illness and the quality and strength of the herbs being used. These are all-important considerations, especially if you're using stronger, more potent herbs in a child's formula.

Suggested Dosages for Children

When Adult Dose is 1 Cup (8 Oz.)

AGE	DOSAGE
Younger than 2 years	½ to 1 teaspoon
2 to 4 years	2 teaspoons
4 to 7 years	1 tablespoon
7 to 11 years	2 tablespoons

When Adult Dose is 1 Teaspoon, or 60 Grains/Drops

AGE	DOSAGE
Younger than 3 months	2 grains/drops
3 to 6 months	3 grains/drops
6 to 9 months	4 grains/drops
9 to 12 months	5 grains/drops
12 to 18 months	7 grains/drops
18 to 24 months	8 grains/drops
2 to 3 years	10 grains/drops
3 to 4 years	12 grains/drops
4 to 6 years	15 grains/drops
6 to 9 years	24 grains/drops
9 to 12 years	30 grains/drops

DETERMINING DOSAGES BY YOUNG'S AND COWLING'S RULES

These rules for dosage determination rely on mathematical calculations using the child's age.

Young's Rule: Add 12 to the child's age. Divide the child's age by this total. Example: Dosage for a 4-year-old: $4 \div 16 = .25$, or $1/4$ of the adult dosage.

Cowling's Rule: Divide the number of child's next birthday by 24. Example: Dosage for a child who is 3, turning 4 years old: $4 \div 24 = .16$, or $1/6$ of the adult dosage.

Determining Measurements by Simpler's Method

While many people are converting to the metric system, I've reverted to Simpler's method of measuring. Many herbalists choose to use this system because it is extremely simple and very versatile. Throughout this book you'll see measurements referred to as "parts"; for example, 3 parts chamomile, 1 part lemon balm, 2 parts oats. A "part" is a unit of measurement that can be interpreted to mean cups, ounces, pounds, tablespoons, or teaspoons — as long as you use that unit consistently throughout the recipe. The use of the word "part" allows the measurement to be determined in relation to the other ingredients. So, if you use tablespoons in the example above, you would have 3 tablespoons chamomile, 1 tablespoon lemon balm, and 2 tablespoons oats.

How to Make Herbal Preparations

Following are some of my favorite ways to administer herbs to children. These suggestions come from years of observing what children will and will not accept. Each child, of course, is unique, and what is acceptable for one may not work for another. Each age group brings with it a different set of challenges. Be innovative and willing to work with the individual nature of each child.

Herbal Teas

The making of herbal tea is a fine art, but it is also bless-edly simple. There are books written on the subject: how to choose the right accoutrements, the proper invitation to send, how warm to serve the chosen blend. I, too, have filled many pages with the art of making and serving herbal tea. But for simplicity's sake, all you really need is a quart jar with a tight-fitting lid, the selected herbs, and water that has reached the boiling point.

There are many delicious and naturally sweet herbs that can be used to flavor the bitter and less familiar flavors of some of the medicinal herbs. For instance, try adding herbs like stevia (sweet herb), marsh mallow root, licorice root, fennel seed, anise seed, Chinese star anise, mints, hibiscus, cinnamon, or ginger. Teas can also be sweetened by mixing them with fruit juice. Warm apple juice mixed with most teas is very good, especially if you add a stick of cinnamon.

For a medicinal tea to be effective, it must be adminis-tered in small amounts several times daily. For chronic prob-lems, serve the tea three or four times daily. For acute ailments such as colds, fevers, and headaches, have the child take several small sips every half hour until the symp-toms subside. Use the dosage chart on page 25 as a guideline for amounts.

To make a tea, use one to three tablespoons of herb(s) for each cup of water. The herb-to-water ratio varies with the quality of herbs being used, whether the herb is fresh or dried (fresh herbs are used in greater amounts than dried), and how strong you wish the tea to be. There are several methods for making herbal teas:

Infusions are made from the more delicate parts of the plant including the leaves, flowers, and aro-matic parts. Place the herb in a container with a tight-fitting lid, and pour boiling water over it. Steep for 30 to 45 minutes. The length of time you steep and the amount of herb you use will determine the strength of the tea.

Decoctions are made from the more tena-cious parts of the plants such as the roots and bark.

It's a little harder to extract the active constituents from these parts, so a slow simmer (or an overnight infusion) is often required. Place herbs in a small saucepan and cover with cold water. Bring to a slow simmer; cover and continue to simmer for approximately 20 minutes. Again, the length of time you simmer plus the amount of herb used will have a direct effect on the strength of the tea.

Solar and lunar infusions utilize the light of the sun and moon to extract the healing properties of the herbs. This is one of my favorite methods of making herb tea. Sometimes after I've prepared herb tea on my kitchen stove, I'll place it in the moonlight or sunlight to pick up some of the rays. I believe we are children of the sky as well as the Earth and that using these energies in our healing work adds a special touch.

When making solar tea, place herbs and water in a glass jar with a tight-fitting lid. Place directly in the hot sunlight for several hours. For lunar tea, herbs can be placed in an open container (unless there are a lot of night flying bugs around!) and positioned directly in the path of the moonlight. Lunar tea is subtle and magical; it is whispered that fairies love to drink it!

Herb Candy

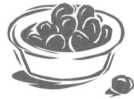

I make a candy I call "jump for joy" balls. They are a favorite way to administer herbs to children (and adults) because they taste delicious and are very effective. The herbs are powdered, then mixed into a paste made with ground fruits and nuts or nut butters and honey. You can flavor herb candy in so many ways. Be creative and invite your children to help you in the process. They'll love their herbal medicine. Just be sure to keep it out of reach.

Once, and only once, I made the mistake of leaving my Super Zoom Balls, a high-energy herbal formula and not a formula for children, on top of the refrigerator. My ambitious and very mischievous grandson managed to maneuver a chair to the counter, climb to the top of the refrigerator and promptly consume half of the herbal candy before he was discovered. Of course, we were all up far longer than we cared to be that night.

To determine the daily dose, it is necessary to know how much powdered herb you included in the total recipe and how many herb balls this amount made. Determine the dosage of herb by using charts provided on pages 25–26. Divide the candy into once-daily dosages.

To make herbal candy:

1. Grind raisins, dates, apricots, and walnuts in a food processor or grinder. Alternatively, you can mix nut butter (such as peanut, almond, or cashew) with honey in equal portions, then proceed with the rest of the steps. *Note:* If you're concerned about the use of honey in small children (due to reports of botulism poisoning), then use maple syrup, rice syrup, or maple cream.
2. Stir in shredded coconut (the unsweetened type found in natural foods stores) and carob powder.
3. Mix in the herb powders well.
4. Roll mixture into balls. Roll again in powdered carob or coconut. Store in refrigerator.

Syrups

Because they are sweet, children often prefer their medicine in syrup form. Syrups are delicious, concentrated extracts of the herbs cooked into a sweet medicine including honey and/or fruit juice. Vegetable glycerin may be substituted for honey. It is an excellent medium for the herbs and is very nutritious.

To make syrup:

1. Use 2 ounces of herb mixture to 1 quart of cold water. Over low heat, simmer the liquid down to 1 pint. This will give you a very concentrated, thick tea.
2. Strain the herbs from the liquid. Compost the herbs and pour the liquid back into the pot.
3. To each pint of liquid, add 1 cup of honey (or other sweetener such as maple syrup, vegetable glycerin, or brown sugar). Most recipes call for 2 cups of sweetener (a 1:1 ratio of sweetener to liquid), but I find it far too sweet. In the days when refrigeration wasn't common, the added sugar helped to preserve the syrup.

4. Warm the honey and liquid together just enough to mix well. Most recipes call for cooking the honey and tea together for 20–30 minutes more, but this method cooks the living enzymes out of the honey.

5. Remove from the heat and bottle for use. You may wish to add a fruit concentrate to flavor, a couple drops of essential oil such as peppermint or spearmint, or a small amount of brandy to help preserve the syrup and aid as a relaxant in cough formulas. Syrups will last for several weeks, even months, if refrigerated.

Herbal Baths

Soothing and calming, an herbal bath can work wonders on a child's nervous system (and the parents' as well). The warm water opens the pores of the skin, the largest organ of elimination and assimilation, and the herbal nutrients flow in. It is like immersing your child in a giant cup of tea.

The temperature of the water will affect the healing quality of the bath. Cool to tepid water is excellent when trying to lower a fever. A warm bath relaxes and soothes the child. My favorite herbs for baby's bath are chamomile, lavender, rose, comfrey, and calendula. To make an herbal bath:

1. Place a handful of herbs in a cotton bag, nylon sock, or strainer and tie on to the nozzle of the tub. Let the hot water run through it for a few minutes.

2. Release the container into the tub and adjust the temperature of the water. Or prepare a strong herbal tea and add the strained tea water to the bathwater.

AN HERBAL BATH FOR A NEWBORN

Herbalists like to say that when Achilles was born, his mother washed him in a bath of warm yarrow tea, knowing that the herb would make her child immortal. But the unbathed spot where she held him was his point of weakness; the infamous achilles' heel, where he would be mortally wounded. So, when giving your newborn his or her first herbal bath anoint every inch of his or her tender new skin.

Herb Powders

Herbs can be powdered and used directly in food and drinks. This is an excellent way to administer herbs to children because it is simple, effective, and the flavor of bitter herbs usually can be masked. It is also easy to regulate the dosage of the herbs being used.

You can powder most herbs in an electric coffee grinder. However, for taste purposes, use separate grinders for your herbs and coffee. Fine herb powders are commercially available. Powdered herbs do not have as long a shelf life as whole herbs, so only powder about ¼ to ½ cup at a time, and store them in airtight glass containers in a dark, cool area or in the refrigerator. Herbal powders can be mixed and matched as needed.

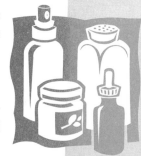

Tinctures

Tinctures are concentrated extracts of herbs. They are taken simply by diluting a few drops of the tincture in warm water or juice. Most tinctures are made with alcohol as the primary solvent or extractant. Though the amount of alcohol is very small, many people choose not to use alcohol-based tinctures for a variety of reasons. Effective tinctures can be made using either vegetable glycerin or apple cider vinegar as the solvent. Though they may not be as strong as alcohol-based preparations, they are perfectly suited to children.

Some of the alcohol in tinctures can be removed by placing the tincture in boiling water for five to ten minutes. This method removes only about 50 percent of the alcohol, however. Since alcoholic tinctures are quite concentrated, it is very important when giving them to children to follow the recommended dosage on the bottle or the guidelines on the dosage chart on page 25. Remember, less is often best.

If choosing alcohol as your solvent, select one that contains 80 to 100 proof alcohol such as vodka, gin, or brandy. Half of the proof number is the percentage of alcohol in the spirits: 80 proof brandy contains 40 percent alcohol, 100 proof vodka contains 50 percent alcohol.

There are several methods used to make tinctures. The traditional or Simpler's method is the one I prefer. It is an extremely simple system that produces beautiful tinctures every time. All that is required to make a tincture in the traditional method are the herbs, the menstruum (alcohol, vinegar, or glycerin base), and a jar with a tight-fitting lid.

To make herbal tinctures:

1. Chop your herbs finely. I recommend using fresh herbs whenever possible. High quality dried herbs will work well also, but one of the advantages of tincturing is the ability to preserve the fresh attributes of the plant. Place the chopped herbs in a clean, dry jar.

2. If using a vegetable glycerin base, dilute it with an equal amount of water before using. If using vinegar as the menstruum, warm the vinegar before pouring it over the herbs (this helps facilitate the release of herbal constituents). Pour the menstruum over the herbs. *Completely cover* the herbs, then add an additional 2–3 inches of liquid. Cover the jar with a tight-fitting lid.

3. Place the jar in a warm, sunny window or other warm place and let the herbs and liquid soak (macerate) for 4–6 weeks. The longer the time, the better. I encourage daily shaking of the tincture bottles during the maceration period. This not only prevents the herbs from packing down on the bottom of the jar, but is also an invitation for some of the old "magic" to come back into medicine making. During the shaking process, you can sing to your tincture jars, stir them in the moonlight or the sunlight, wave feathers over them — whatever your imagination inspires you to do.

4. At the end of the maceration time, strain the herbs from the menstruum. Use a large stainless steel strainer lined with cheesecloth or muslin. Reserve the liquid, which is now a potent tincture, and compost the herbs. Rebottle, label, and store out of the reach of children.

Tinctures have a very long shelf life, almost indefinite, and should be stored in a cool, dark location. Because of their concentration, follow the dosage chart carefully.

GLYCERIN-BASED TINCTURES

Personally, I feel that glycerites (glycerin-based tinctures) are much better suited for children. When properly made, there're quite strong enough. Because of the sweet nature of glycerin, they taste far better than alcohol tinctures. And they have a long shelf life. My dear friend, Sunny Mavor, developed an excellent line of herbal tinctures just for children and made them all with a glycerin base. Her product line, Herbs for Kids, can be found in most health foods stores.

Herbal Pops

These herbal popsicles are a fun and easy way to get a child to take his or her prescribed tea formula. Herbal pops are refreshing in the summertime and provide the wonderful healing properties of the herbs in a delicious and fun form. Because they are so cold, I do not recommend them for cold types of imbalances such as flu, colic, ear infections, or respiratory infections. The cold makes them excellent for teething babies, however. You may be very creative with these pops, and include flowers and herbs in the frozen cubes for beauty and fun.

To make herbal pops:
1. Make a strong tea following the directions on page 27, but triple the amount of herb to water. Strain.
2. Dilute with an equal amount of apple juice or any other favorite juice. Pour into popsicle trays; freeze.

Herbal Enemas

A warm catnip enema will bring down a child's fever and provide necessary fluid to the system in extreme cases when the child cannot keep down fluids. It is an excellent way to administer the healing essences of herbs into a sick and feverish body. Though unfamiliar to most people these days, enemas are a time-tested home remedy. They should not be used in children under 3 years of age unless recommended by a holistic health care practioner or pediatrician.

It is absolutely essential that one be experienced at administering an enema correctly. If you've never given this treatment before, consult your pediatrician or holistic health care provider for instructions. Do not use this treatment unless recommended by your health care professional.

To prepare an herbal enema:

1. Following the directions on page 27 make 1 pint of catnip tea using 3 tablespoons of herb per pint of water. Heat very slowly over low heat for 15 minutes.

2. Remove from heat and let cool to proper temperature. Use a cool, but not cold, enema to lower fevers. Strain well and pour less than 1 cup of liquid into an enema bag.

3. Place enema bag at shoulder height so that liquid can flow smoothly. Lubricate the tip with herbal salve or oil and insert into the rectum. *Slowly* release a gentle flow of liquid. Use an enema bag that lets you regulate the flow of liquid and be sure the flow is gentle and slow.

You would be wise to have the child in a tub during this process. The longer the child holds the liquid in the more effective the enema. But even if the child holds the liquid in for just a couple of minutes, the medicine will be effective. It is helpful, after withdrawing the tip, to fold a towel and press firmly over the anus for a few minutes to aid in retention.

ADMINISTERING HERBAL MEDICINE TO INFANTS

Mother's milk is the most effective and safest way to administer herbs to infants. It is necessary for the mother to drink at least four to six cups of the tea daily. Not only will the baby have the benefits of the gentle healing herbs, but the mother will as well. If a mother is not nursing, herbal teas and tinctures can be added directly to the young one's bottle.

chapter four

Herbal Remedies for Common Childhood Ailments

By closely observing your child, you can usually detect when he or she is stressed, anxious, or out of balance, and thus more susceptible to illness. Illness rarely just occurs. Usually it is a result of a stressed immune system, emotional imbalance, lack of sleep, poor hygiene, or poor nutrition.

Sometimes illness occurs because the child is just having too much fun whirling through life. Dr. Hans Selye, the man who popularized the word "stress," defined it as a nonspecific response of the body to external stimuli — anything from the lash of whip to a passionate kiss. Children live in passion, and the great abundance of energy required to maintain such high levels of activity can leave even the most exuberant of spirits exhausted and depleted.

All children are born with inherent strengths and weaknesses. Watch for these patterns early in life. Pay close attention to the energy levels of your child. Observe him or her through the seasons, noting which season brings with it its own special challenges for your child. Note when and to what he or she is most susceptible. This will help you become more aware of your child's health patterns.

This information is shared in the spirit that it may assist you in helping your child through the illnesses of childhood. It is not meant to replace the professional advice of a holistic health care provider or a family physician, but rather to complement such advice.

Teething

Unavoidable, teething affects all children, with varying degrees of discomfort. Though not an illness, it generally is a time of great frustration for both parent and child — for parents because it seems no matter how hard they try they can't remove the pain and thus feel helpless; for the child because he or she is experiencing one of the early pains of life and it hurts!

Often when a child has difficulty teething, various symptoms will arise. Intermittent fever, diaper and other rashes, extreme crankiness, and diarrhea are not uncommon. Treat each symptom appropriately following the guidelines suggested in this book, but remember that support is the primary lesson called for here. The teething process is natural, like many of the other life cycles we'll go through in a lifetime. It marks the child's first experience of "biting in," her ability to deal with the stress of life, to call on her own powers as well as the support of family and friends. Rather than isolating or protecting the child, support and reassure her (along with yourself, if needed) that this is a natural process. Thousands of human babies have gone through this before, and yours can too. The rewards will be a shining set of healthy teeth, and the ability to enjoy another of life's great pleasures: the art of good eating.

Catnip Tea

This is an old standby for both child and parent during the teething times. Catnip is soothing to the nervous system and helps to relieve acute pain. It is also helpful for teething-related fevers. Administer as tea or tincture in frequent small doses. The tea itself is not tasty, so you may wish to formulate with other gentle nervines such as chamomile, roses, passionflower, or lemon balm. Dr. Jethro Kloss, a famous herbalist and doctor of the early 1900s, spoke impassionately of catnip: "If every mother would have catnip on her shelf, it would save her many a sleepless night and her child much suffering." It was particularly thoughtful of him to consider the mother and, following his advice, I always suggest catnip and passionflower tea for the parents of teething children.

High Calcium Tea

This blend is very helpful for all ages to give to the child throughout the teething period. It is most effective if it is given several weeks or even months before teething begins. It supplies necessary calcium in a form that the body can easily digest and assimilate; use it to supplement a natural diet rich in calcium.

An excellent blend of herbs that add high quality, naturally biochelated calcium and other important minerals to the diet, High Calcium Tea is also good for children during growth spurts, and when there is any bone or muscle injury.

High Calcium Tea

1 part nettle	3 parts rose hips
2 parts oats	½ part cinnamon
1 part raspberry leaf	a pinch of stevia to
2 parts lemongrass	sweeten (optional)
2 parts lemon balm	

Combine herbs and store in an airtight container. Make a tea following the directions on page 27. Use the dosage chart on page 25 to determine the amount used.

Rose Hip Syrup

Giving frequent doses of Rose Hip Syrup can often relieve teething symptoms. Give four to six drops of Rose Hip Syrup every hour for infants. For older children give 100 to 200 mg vitamin C in acerola tablets daily along with frequent teaspoon doses of Rose Hip Syrup. Follow the directions on page 29 to make an herbal syrup.

CALCIUM SUPPLEMENTS

Most calcium tablets are difficult to digest and are expensive substances that your body must find a way to eliminate. There are some fine natural calcium supplements on the market. They usually have low dosages of calcium and are made of 100 percent natural food substances such as sesame seeds, dark green leafy vegetables, sea vegetables, and herbs. Take your reading glasses along with you even to the natural foods store and inspect those labels carefully, especially the small print.

Hyland Teething Tablets

Hyland Homeopathic Pharmacy makes a wonderful herbal teething tablet for children. Interestingly, most parents have reported that although the teething formula Hyland's manufactures works well, the formula for colic is even more effective for teething babies. So I generally recommend Hyland's colic formula for teething difficulties. Try both and let me know which works better for you.

Herbal Pops

Frozen catnip or chamomile pops are excellent for teething children to suck on. The cold helps numb the gums and relieves the pain. Children generally love these pops and they'll suck intently on them until the pain subsides and they're gurgling away happily again.

Clove Oil

Though clove oil is often recommended for sore gums and tooth decay, I generally do not recommend it for teething babies; the oil is far too strong for a child's mouth. If you decide to use it because nothing else is working, then dilute it in a vegetable oil base: 1 drop of essential oil of clove to ½ ounce of olive (or any other vegetable) oil. Test it on your own gums. Remember that your gums are much less sensitive than babies' gums. You should barely feel it. Massage gently into the gum area. It can be comforting to a teething baby; it will numb the area and help relieve any inflammation. *Never let children put clove oil on their own gums and always use it highly diluted.*

Colic

Colic, a term used to describe an infant's tummy ache, can be a heart-wrenching experience for both the parents and the infant. It is generally caused by painful spasmodic contractions of the infant's immature digestive tract or by air and gas trapped in the intestines. The digestive tract of an infant generally takes about three months to mature. This is the time period in which most colic clears up.

Depending on the degree of sensitivity, mealtimes can be a painful ordeal. Generally, with a little patience, some simple dietary changes, and the addition of a few gentle, time-tested herbal remedies, even the most persistent colic clears up or is, at least, lessened.

However, I recently encountered my first colic cure failure! A dear friend and herbal apprentice had just had her first baby. But shortly after birth, Dylan developed one of the worst cases of infant colic I have ever witnessed. His parents tried every remedy and suggestion offered by well-meaning friends, parents, their herbal community, and their fellow churchgoers. Nothing seemed to work. Fortunately, after several months, the colic disappeared as mysteriously as it came. Dylan is now the epitome of cheerfulness, and his tummy aches are gone. Once again, the lesson here seems to be that support is something we all need every time we go through a life process.

The following suggestions are all gentle and effective and work in harmony with the sensitive nature of the infant.

Create a Relaxed Environment

Often colicky children are extremely sensitive to their environment. Since you, the parent, *are* a child's primary environment and source of emotional and physical nourishment, your well-being can contribute to the presence or absence of colic. Quiet, peaceful music during mealtimes is often helpful. Mothers should drink warm nervine teas before nursing. Feeding time should, whenever possible, be a time of quiet, restful sharing. Turn off the TV; whatever is being aired is part of the feeding process for your baby. If you are feeling stressed out and tense, the infant will often respond with similar energy. This does not mean that all colicky babies have stressed-out parents, but it is important to note that a peaceful environment is conducive to creating well-being for the child.

Avoid Irritating Foods

If nursing, mothers should avoid foods that are irritating to the infant's digestive tract. While every child's system is different, some foods are common digestive-tract irritants. The brassica family, which includes cabbage, broccoli, cauliflower, kale, and collards, is high in sulfur, which creates gas in the intestines. Avoid hot, spicy foods; an infant's system just isn't ready for them yet. And avoid chocolate, peanuts, peanut butter, and foods high in sugar. Such foods slow down digestive action, cause congestion in the digestive tract, and add to the spasms and contractions of colic. Regularly monitor your child to determine which foods are irritating to him/her.

Though the amount of caffeine in your daily coffee may not seem to directly affect you anymore, it is nonetheless a powerful stimulant. Your child's young system will respond readily to this common drug's stimulating properties and she may become nervous and highly excitable. Coffee is also very acidic and will adversely affect the immature digestive system of the infant, adding to the difficulties of colic.

Supplement with Acidophilus

Acidophilus or Bacillus Bifidus is highly recommended for infant colic. They are naturally occurring flora found in the human intestines, and supplements will help build up healthy intestinal flora and support the growth of digestive enzymes. There are special preparations of each of these substances for children, available in most natural foods stores. Be sure you get an active, viable form of acidophilus. I generally recommend Natrin, a brand name that seems to be consistently good. To treat colic, double the amount suggested on the label. A standard dose for colic would be ¼ teaspoon four to five times daily.

If the child is eating solid foods and is not lactose-intolerant, include daily servings of yogurt, kefir, and buttermilk, which contain acidophilus. If nursing, the mother should eat several servings a day of these foods.

Herbal Teas

The most helpful herbs for treating colic are slippery elm, fennel, anise, dill, and catnip. Try these teas to relieve the acute symptoms of colic.

Slippery Elm Gruel

This gruel (thick tea) is wonderfully soothing and healing. It is also extremely nourishing. Since the herbs are in powder form, there's no need to strain this gruel. Slippery elm and marsh mallow root are both extremely mucilaginous. This makes them very soothing and healing to the intestinal tract, but very difficult to strain. If, however, you choose to strain the gruel, line a large strainer with cheesecloth, pour the tea into it, and let it slowly drain through. When cool enough to handle, gather up the cheesecloth and squeeze the remaining gruel through.

> 1 part slippery elm bark, powdered
> 1 part marsh mallow root, powdered
> ⅛ part cinnamon, powdered
> ⅛ part fennel seed, powdered
> maple syrup to taste

1. Combine first four ingredients and store in an airtight container until ready to use.
2. Combine 1 tablespoon of herb mixture and 1 cup of boiling water in a pan. Cover, and cook over low heat for 10–15 minutes. Sweeten with maple syrup.
3. Store the liquid in the refrigerator; warm before serving. The tea can be mixed with juice or in cereal. The infant may drink as much of this tea as desired. If nursing, the mother should drink 3–4 cups daily.

Seed Tea

Dill and anise were at one time such favorite herbs for colic that English nursery rhymes were written in honor of them. Seed Tea helps to expel gas and relieve the symptoms of colic.

> 1 part fennel   3 parts chamomile
> 1 part dill   ¼ part catnip
> 3 parts anise   a pinch of stevia to sweeten

1. Mix ingredients and store in an airtight container until ready to use.

2. Infuse 1 tablespoon mixture in 1 cup boiling water and let sit, covered, for 45 minutes. Cool and strain.

3. Give the infant teaspoon dosages every few minutes until colic pain ceases. This tea may also be given effectively in small doses before feeding time. ⌇

Colic Tablets

Hyland Pharmacy has a homeopathic colic tablet that is very good. It is available in most natural foods stores. A safe, all-natural product, this old-time remedy has provided relief for countless colicky babies. Follow the dosage outlined on the bottle.

Old-Fashioned Techniques That Still Work

In the midst of a colic attack, there are a couple of old-fashioned and effective techniques to try. Place your baby in a warm chamomile or lavender bath. If bottle-fed, the baby can enjoy his feeding from the comfort of this soothing bath. You may relax the child's stomach muscles by placing a towel that was soaked in hot herb tea — such as chamomile or lavender — over the stomach area. Be certain the towel is adequately warm, but not hot. The combination of warm water and herbal essence will often be just what's needed to stop the muscle spasms. A drop or two of lavender or chamomile essential oil in the bath water or on the towel will often work wonders.

And there is always the old reliable burping technique. Pad your shoulder and place the child's head against it. Pat his or her back gently. Children seem to become hypnotized into forgetting the problem. What is really happening, of course, along with distracting the child from his grief for a few moments, is that you are helping to move the gas deposits along with a steady movement.

Cradle Cap

Neither a serious nor contagious problem, a child will usually outgrow cradle cap in time. The sebaceous glands of most infants are not developed and may oversecrete, causing a yellowish, oily crust on the child's scalp. You can remove the "cap" and help regulate the activity of the sebaceous glands by gently massaging a mixture of herbs and olive oil into the scalp two or three times daily. Leave the herb/oil mixture on overnight. The next morning the crust can be easily removed by gently massaging. Be sure not to pick at the scab or be too rough. Shampoo with a mild baby shampoo only when necessary.

Tea for Cradle Cap

If cradle cap continues to be persistent, give the infant this warm herbal tea.

> 1 part red clover flower
> 1 part burdock root
> 1 part mullein leaf

1. Mix herbs and store in an airtight container until ready to use.
2. Add 1 cup boiling water to 1 teaspoon of herb mixture and steep for 30 minutes. Strain.
3. Give the infant 2 teaspoons of the tea 3–4 times daily for several weeks. 🌀

Cradle Cap Oil

> 1 part dried nettle leaf
> 1 part chamomile flowers
> 1 part mullein leaf
> olive oil
> lavender essential oil

1. In a double boiler, combine herbs. Cover with olive oil. Cook over very low heat for about 1 hour. Strain, and bottle.
2. Add 1 drop of lavender essential oil to each ounce of herbal oil. Store in a cool area or the refrigerator. Oil should always be at room temperature before application. 🌀

Diaper Rash

Most diaper rashes respond readily to natural therapy. Follow the suggestions listed with good faith; all have been used successfully by countless mothers. If the diaper rash is persistent and does not respond to natural therapies, it could be a herpes-related virus or yeast-type fungus. Consult your holistic health care practitioner or pediatrician in such cases.

One or more of the following irritants generally causes diaper rashes:

- **Harsh, irritating detergents** can leave a soap residue on the diapers. Simply change soaps. Use mild soap flakes such as Ivory or a liquid soap such as Heavenly Horsetail or Basic H. Do not use detergents or ammonia, and never use bleach. As harmful as bleach is for the environment, it is even worse for your baby.
- **Irritating foods** affect the child's digestive system. Spicy foods, citrus fruits, and other high-acid foods are major irritants and can affect the child both when eaten directly and through the mother's milk.
- **Teething, fever, and other stress-related incidents** cause toxins to be released in the child's system, which can sometimes be manifested as diaper rashes or other skin-related problems.

Give Acidophilus Preparations

Administer ¼ teaspoon acidophilus culture (available in natural foods stores) 3 times daily. Use a preparation that's formulated especially for children. You can even try spreading acidophilus diluted in plain unsweetened yogurt directly on the rash.

Take Off Those Diapers!

Leave diapers off as much as possible. The more exposure to air and sunlight the better, though you must be sure to protect your child's delicate skin from sunburn. If the weather is uncooperative or the diaper rash persists, consider using an herbal preparation. Prolonged or recurrent diaper rash should be examined by a pediatrician or holistic practioner.

Much of the time when my son was growing up, we lived in the mountains, as close to nature as possible. He seldom wore diapers — or any clothes, for that matter — as there was simply no reason to, and the less I had to wash the happier I was. Jason never once had a diaper rash. He does, however, have a stigma about nakedness, and I wonder if it isn't a result of his wayward mom's habits.

Herbal Powders

Use arrowroot powder or a special clay/herb mix for your baby powder and as a remedy for diaper rash. Cornstarch, an old-fashioned remedy, is also very effective but is not recommended for use on yeast-related diaper rashes, as it may encourage the growth of certain bacteria. Commercial baby powder is made with talc, which is a possible carcinogen. It also contains synthetic scents, which can be irritating to an infant's sensitive skin. Make your own baby powder (see page 69) or buy those that are made with natural ingredients. Take care not to disperse the powder too much around babies who have respiratory problems.

Herbal Salve

An herbal salve made with St.-John's-wort, comfrey leaf and root, and calendula (see recipe on page 68) is one of the

COVERING BABY'S BOTTOM

Use only 100 percent cotton diapers and change after every bowel movement. Rinse the baby's bottom frequently and dry thoroughly.

If your child is prone to diaper rash, you may choose to do away with plastic pants, a prime contributor to rashes (not to mention landfills). Instead, use a natural wool soaker. These are nonirritating, highly absorbent, and widely available. Denise, my grandson's mother, made all of her own cloth diapers and wool soakers for Andrew. He had the cutest ones on the block. And, again, never a diaper rash in his entire infancy or toddler stage.

best remedies I know of for diaper rash. This is a famous old-time formula that I've been making for more than 25 years. It still remains one of the best recipes out there and is a superior remedy for diaper rashes.

Wash and dry the baby's bottom after each bowel movement, apply the herbal salve, and follow with a light dusting of clay/herb powder. This treatment plan used in conjunction with the other suggestions listed will generally clear up the worst diaper rash, unless herpes or staph is involved.

Herbal Paste

For a more serious rash, mix the clay/herb powder with water or a tea of comfrey to form a thin paste. Smooth over rash and leave on for 30 to 45 minutes. To remove, gently rinse with warm water or soak off in a warm tub. Don't attempt to scrape or peel the paste off, as you may further injure the child's irritated skin.

Diarrhea

There are few children who have not had a bout of diarrhea, or it's counterpart, constipation. Diarrhea can be caused by a number of problems, the most common being reactions to or excesses of certain food groups, reactions to bacteria and viruses, teething, fever, emotional upset, or an infection elsewhere in the body.

The primary concern with diarrhea is dehydration, which can occur quickly if fluid intake is not being carefully monitored, and can be fatal if severe. Ensure that the child's fluid intake is adequate. Don't just guess; monitor the amount of liquid the child drinks and give him warm baths. These will help in the absorption of liquid.

Though liquid intake is essential, it is not necessary that the child eat solid food. It is actually best if they only consume liquids such as herb teas, vegetable broth, and chicken or miso soup. Eating solid food will make the already stressed digestive system work overtime. It also means more runny diapers, as everything eaten will quickly come out. If the child wishes to eat, allow foods such as yogurt, kefir, buttermilk, cottage cheese, potato soup, mashed potatoes (no gravy or butter), and slippery elm gruel (see recipe on page 42). These foods are easy to digest and will contribute to healing the irritated digestive system. Though milk products will often exacerbate diarrhea, cultured milk products such as buttermilk and yogurt add beneficial bacteria that aid the system. Also, administer ⅛ teaspoon of acidophilus culture every hour until diarrhea stops. In addition, commercial pediatric electrolyte solutions, such as Pedialyte, are very helpful in preventing dehydration.

Blackberry Root Tea

Along with a high fluid intake, herbal baths, and a very simple diet as suggested above, this tea should help remedy diarrhea. Unfortunately, and for reasons I've never fathomed, blackberry root tincture is hard to find. You may have to make your own. It's simple:

> 1 part dry or fresh blackberry root, finely chopped
> alcohol or vegetable glycerin
> ½ cup warm water

Follow the directions for making a tincture on page 32. Mix 1 teaspoon of tincture in ½ cup warm water and administer ¼ teaspoon of this preparation every hour. 🌱

Diarrhea Remedy Tea

To make this tea more palatable, you can add a small amount of maple syrup or blackberry juice concentrate (available in natural foods stores) for flavor.

> 3 parts blackberry root
> 2 parts slippery elm bark
> ⅛ part cinnamon

Mix herbs and store in an airtight container. Simmer 1 teaspoon of the herb mixture in 1 cup water for 20 minutes. Strain and cool. Administer 2–4 tablespoons every hour, or more often as needed. 🌱

Constipation

Constipation is frequently associated with emotional factors or habits learned at an early age that do not support healthy elimination. Be critical of such behavior when assessing your child's toilet habits. Catching the problem early may eliminate a lifetime of stressful elimination. Constipation is one of the most common problems adults suffer; witness the number of products in any drug store that have been developed for a constipated society. Often, simple habits learned early will eliminate the need for stronger medications later on. Children experience constipation for the same reasons adults do. How many adults do you know who can't go to the bathroom because they don't have the time, or they are unfamiliar with the bathroom, or are made to feel insecure and uncomfortable?

If your child develops constipation, the first step is to avoid foods that contribute to the problem. High-fat dairy foods, cheese, wheat, eggs, and refined, processed foods are generally the most common food culprits; watch your child for signs of constipation after consuming these foods. If the child is nursing, the mother should avoid these foods in her diet as well, until the constipation clears up. If the child is bottle-fed on cow's milk, switch to goat's milk or soy milk. Cow's milk can be constipating to some children as well as adults.

Include in the diet those foods that contribute to good elimination: fruits, vegetables, whole grains, liquids, molasses, dried fruit, and foods that supply bulk to the system. There are several herbs that should be included in the child's diet when needed: carob powder, slippery elm, flaxseed, psyllium seed, licorice root, and Irish moss. These plants can be powdered in a coffee grinder and added to the child's meals. Use 1 to 4 teaspoons 3 to 4 times daily, or as often as needed during constipation. For children under 10, use the smaller dose. These herbs are not laxative herbs per se, but provide necessary bulk in the diet.

The following suggestions combined with the dietary recommendations should bring relief to the child plagued by constipation:

- Administer ½ teaspoon child's acidophilus with meals. Acidophilus adds friendly bacteria to the digestive tract and aids in good digestion.
- Grind equal amounts of slippery elm, flaxseed, and psyllium seed together until finely powdered. Mix 1 teaspoon of the mixture in with food at each meal.
- Make a special "candy" by grinding prunes, figs, apricots, and raisins together. Mix in powdered psyllium seed, slippery elm, and fennel seed. To flavor and thicken, mix in carob powder, which is made from an herb that's useful for treating constipation. Roll into balls and serve daily as a delicious, nourishing snack.
- Be sure the child drinks plenty of room temperature water. When constipated, upon rising give the child a cup of warm psyllium seed water (soak 1 teaspoon of psyllium seed in 1 cup of water overnight. Add lemon juice to taste).
- Exercise is critical for regular bowel movements. For most children, exercise is not a problem, but you may choose to make a regular time to do some activities together. A nice morning walk is a good way to get the energy moving and is also a nice opportunity to spend time together. The primary goal is to provide some centered, peaceful activity that moves the body while relaxing the mind and spirit.

Tea for Constipation

1 part marsh mallow root	1 part licorice root
2 parts psyllium seed	¼ part orange peel
4 parts fennel seed	½ part cinnamon
2 parts spearmint	a pinch of stevia

Combine all ingredients and store in an airtight container. In a saucepan over low heat, simmer 1 teaspoon herb mixture in 1 cup boiling water for 20 minutes. Strain and allow to cool. Administer ⅛–½ cup tea with meals or as often as needed. If constipation persists, add ⅛ part senna pod or leaf to the recipe.

Earaches

Until a child is three or four years old, the ear canals are not fully formed and, consequently, do not drain well. When a child gets congested or has a cold, the ear canals get plugged up with excess mucus, which then cannot drain properly. Bacteria begin to grow in the moisture of the accumulated secretions and infection often occurs.

Ear infections can result from allergies. If your child has recurring ear infections despite your best efforts, consider the possibility of allergies. Wheat, citrus, and dairy products, including milk, cheese, and ice cream, are the most common offenders. If allergies are suspect, don't despair. There are effective natural remedies for allergies.

Ear infections can be serious. Treated improperly, they can leave a child with impaired hearing or permanently deaf. It is important to treat an ear infection at the first sign of the infection and to work in conjunction with a holistic health care practitioner and your family pediatrician. Watch for the early signs: congestion, colds, runny nose, fever, excessive rubbing or pulling of the ear lobe, combined with irritability and fussiness. If your child wakes up screaming in the night and pulling at her ears, an infection has eked its way into the ear canals and will need to be attended to immediately.

The use of antibiotics, though sometimes effective for acute situations, does not correct the cause of the problem. Because antibiotics (which means "against life") can create such havoc in the young child's system, disrupting the immune cycle and making one further susceptible to disease, it is important whenever using antibiotics to follow the suggestions outlined in this section.

In addition, when a child has an ear infection, be sure to avoid giving her any congesting type foods: eggs, dairy, wheat, sugar, orange juice, and all refined, processed foods.

Rest and Simple Remedies

It is imperative that a child with an ear infection gets plenty of rest and does not go out into the cold air prematurely. It is a common mistake to think a child has recovered from an ear infection and send him out to play. So many times have I heard that "Johnny kept me awake crying all night with a bad ear infection. Come morning, he was fine so I sent him off to school. But, wouldn't you know it, that ear infection was back in full force again in the middle of the night." Ear infections have a way of doing that. Usually, what happens is that the child is just happy to be feeling better and wants to get out and play. Seriously consider keeping the child housebound for at least a few days until recovery is complete.

Acidophilus culture, given in doses of ½ teaspoon several times daily, can be very helpful for ear infections. Also try a tasty tea of fresh grated ginger, fresh squeezed lemons, and honey or maple syrup. It is a refreshing, decongesting blend.

Be certain the child's kidneys are working well and he is taking in sufficient fluid. Warm packs placed over the lower back (the area of the kidneys) can help relieve ear infections. This technique stems from traditional Chinese medicine, in which the health of the kidneys is directly connected to the health of the ears. Note, however, that this treatment should be combined with other therapies for optimal results. Cranberry juice is a strengthening tonic for the kidneys. As prevention during cold weather, children prone to ear infections should wear hats with earflaps and the area of the kidneys should be kept warm.

Garlic and Mullein Flower Oil

One of the best herbal remedies for ear infections. It is important to treat both ears; the ear canals are connected and the infection can move back and forth. The oil not only helps fight the infection, but also relieves the pain. Be absolutely sure the oil is warm, not hot.

2–3 tablespoons mullein flowers (fresh flowers are best, but dried flowers may be used)
2–3 tablespoons chopped garlic
olive oil

1. Place the garlic and mullein flowers in a double boiler or small saucepan. Add just enough olive oil to cover the herbs. Over very low heat, warm for 20–30 minutes.
2. Strain well and store in a tightly covered glass jar in the refrigerator. I generally strain through a fine wire mesh strainer lined with cheesecloth.
3. To use, warm the oil in a teaspoon held over a candle or stove top. Warm *only* to the temperature of mother's milk (about room temperature).
4. Suction oil into a dropper and instill several drops into the ear. Administer the warm herbal oil every 30 minutes or as often as needed. Any extra oil will drain out on its own within a few minutes. ✿

Tincture for Infections

The herbs in this recipe can also be powdered and capsulated to administer to older children.

¼ part organically grown goldenseal root
1 part echinacea root
1 part usnea
1 part garlic (fresh)
¼ part gingerroot

Follow the directions on page 32 for making a tincture. Administer ⅛ teaspoon of the tincture diluted in warm water or juice orally 3 times daily. ✿

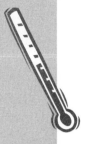

Fevers

Fevers of themselves are a natural mechanism to rid the body of infection and are the sign of a healthy immune system. It is only when the fever gets too high or lingers too long that it can be debilitating, even devastating. If your child's fever reaches 102°F or more or lasts for several days, contact your holistic health care provider or pediatrician immediately.

With small children, it is imperative to keep fluid intake high. Dehydration is the greatest danger of childhood fevers, not the actual temperature of a fever.

Use the following techniques for lowering and controlling a child's fever.

Apple Cider Vinegar Treatments

To lower a fever, bathe the child in a tepid bath. Mix ¼ cup apple cider vinegar into the tub. Be certain there are no drafts in the room. After the bath, quickly wrap the child in a warm flannel sheet. Placing a drop or two of diluted pure chamomile essential oil on the sheet is very helpful.

Another treatment is to wrap the child's feet in a cool cloth that has been dipped in a mixture of apple cider vinegar and water. Keep the child bundled warmly.

Fever Reducing Tea

- 2 parts catnip
- 2 parts elder blossoms
- 1 part peppermint
- 1 part echinacea root

Mix herbs and store in an airtight container. Add 1 cup boiling water to 1 teaspoon of the mixture and steep for 1 hour. Administer every 30 minutes. See dosage chart on page 25 for guidelines. 🌱

Chicken Pox, Measles, and Other Skin Eruptions

Though chicken pox and measles are distinctly different, treatment is similar. When treating these common disorders of childhood, you want to aid the body's natural defense mechanisms. Though these illnesses are a great discomfort for the child, most children sail right through them. My son, Jason, avoided these "natural" childhood illnesses. I'd dutifully take him around the neighborhood exposing him whenever possible, knowing that the earlier a child gets these illnesses the better able he is to cope with it. But his immune system seemed resistant to them and, to my suprise, he never got them.

The following treatments are geared toward helping the body's natural immunity and its inherent ability to respond to these childhood disorders. However, be sure to involve your pediatrician if the child is under 2 years old, and always treat measels more cautiously.

Super Immunity Syrup

This formula can also be made into a tea, but you'll need to add some pleasant tasting herbs such as lemon balm and lemongrass for flavor. Super Immunity Syrup helps assist the body in warding off infection, and lessens the uncomfortable effects of the rash.

> 1 part echinacea root and tops
> 1 part astragalus root
> 2 parts oats (milky green tops)
> 1 part burdock root

Follow the directions for making herbal syrups on page 29. At the onset of infection, administer 1 teaspoon every hour until symptoms clear. Use 4–6 times daily during the course of an infection. 🌱

Tea for Chicken Pox and Measles

- 1 part calendula
- 1 part red clover
- 2 parts oats (milky tops)
- 2 parts lemon balm
- 1 part passionflower

Mix herbs and store in an airtight container. Add 1 cup boiling water to 1 teaspoon mixture and steep for 30 minutes. Strain, sweeten with stevia, honey, or maple syrup. Let the child drink as much as desired. 🌿

Valerian-Burdock Tincture for Itching and Skin Rash

This is my favorite formula to help relieve itching and promote relaxation. You can purchase burdock, echinacea, and valerian tinctures ready-made from most natural foods stores. Mix together 2 parts of burdock root to 1 part valerian and 1 part echinacea.

- 2 parts burdock root
- 1 part echinacea root
- 1 part valerian root

Make a tincture as instructed on page 32. Give ⅛ teaspoon tincture (or see chart on page 25) every 2 hours.

For some children, valerian acts as a stimulant. If you notice your child becoming more irritated and active after using it, discontinue immediately. 🌿

Oatmeal Bath

Nothing's as soothing to itchy, irritated skin as a warm oatmeal bath. For extra comfort, place the strained oatmeal in a cotton bag or sock and add it to the bathwater. A couple of drops of lavender oil, in addition to being a relaxing nervine, has antibacterial and disinfectant properties.

Prepare a big pot of oatmeal, adding three times as much water as usual. Cook for five minutes. Strain. Add the liquid to the bathwater.

Disinfectant Powder

Mix up this herbal powder and keep on hand as a disinfectant. It can be sprinkled directly on oozing pox sores, helping to dry them as well as preventing infection from setting in. You may also try sprinkling slippery elm powder over the sores. It's so soothing and helps to stop the itching.

- 1 ounce green clay (available from natural foods and herb stores)
- 1 tablespoon comfrey root powder
- 1 tablespoon calendula flower, powdered
- ½ tablespoon cultivated goldenseal or chaparral powder

Combine all ingredients. Sprinkle on skin sores to stop itching and promote drying. Store remaining powder in a shaker container or glass bottle with a tight-fitting lid. ✺

TO PREVENT SCRATCHING AND SCARRING

If a sick child is suffering from itching and is scratching frequently, put socks on the child's hands, especially at night, to prevent him from injuring the skin. A gentle but strong herbal nervine tea or tincture such as skullcap, valerian, or catnip is also recommended.

Vitamin E can be used both topically and internally to prevent scarring. Prick open one end of a 1,000 I.U. capsule and apply the oil directly to the injured area before scars have formed. For internal use, give 50 I.U. to 100 I.U. twice daily, depending on the age of the child.

Rescue Remedy Flower Essence Spritzer

Try spraying this spritzer in a child's room to relieve stress and anxiety.

    3 ½ ounces distilled water
      3 drops lavender essential oil
      4 drops Rescue Remedy (Five-Flower Remedy)
      1 tablespoon brandy

Combine all ingredients in a 4-ounce spritzer bottle with a mister top. Shake before using. Use as a room spray as needed. ✺

Colds and Flus

There's probably not a child alive who has escaped childhood without at least a cold or two. Unless these all too common maladies are reccurring, there's no need for concern. The various "bugs" and viruses that cause colds and flus allow the immune system to kick into action and do its job. These illnesses also provide the opportunity for us to observe how quickly our bodies respond to common illness, and they serve as indicators of our overall health.

Lots of fluids, warm soup, a couple days of rest, and a few specific herbal remedies along with some immune-

USING FLOWER ESSENCES

Flower essences, available at most natural foods stores, are gentle healing remedies made from the flowers of plants. They are some of the most helpful remedies for children, and in times of stress they seem to work miracles. Flower essences can be used in conjunction with any type of medication without causing complications or side effects. Try adding Rescue Remedy (sometimes called Five-Flower Remedy) to the bathwater, or give a drop or two under the child's tongue several times daily. This remedy produces a calming, centering feeling and is excellent during times of stress and trauma.

strengthening herbs are generally all that's needed. If your child continues to get colds and flus or is having difficulty recovering from a particularly devastating flu, then seek the guidance of a holistic health care provider or your family doctor.

At the first sign of a cold or flu, start giving your child frequent, higher than normal doses of echinacea tincture. For example, a child of four would take ⅛ teaspoon of echinacea tincture every hour until the symptoms subside.

Super Immune Tincture

Though echinacea is often effective by itself, a stronger immune support tincture may be used instead of or in addition to the echinacea. Here is a favorite formula.

    2 parts echinacea (root, leaves, and flowers)
    1 part usnea
    2 parts licorice root
    ½ part garlic
    ½ part lomatium root
    ½ part reishi mushroom

Combine herbs and store in an airtight container. Prepare a tincture as described on page 32. This tincture will not taste good, so dilute with juice or herb tea, or mix with fruit juice concentrate to help flavor it. See chart on page 25 for dosage.

VITAMIN C THERAPY

Another tactic I've found helpful in fighting colds and flus is to give high doses (up to 5,000 milligrams) of vitamin C, usually in liquid form, to the child. Start with a smaller dose, and increase gradually. If the child develops runny stools, decrease the amount. High doses of vitamin C do seem to help kick the immune response into action. It works best at the onset of colds and flus, helping to prevent or lessen the symptoms.

Elderberry Syrup

This is the most popular herbal cold remedy in Europe, and it's delicious. Every year I try to make two or three batches of Elderberry Syrup, and it's always gone by the end of the season. I've gathered fresh elderberries from the West Coast to the East Coast and have marked the seasons by the ripening of these dark blue/black berries. Use only blue elderberries; the red ones are potentially toxic if eaten in large quantities. Never eat elderberries that haven't been cooked first.

> 1 cup fresh or ½ cup dried elderberries
> 3 cups water
> 1 cup honey

Place the berries in a saucepan and cover with water. Simmer over low heat for 30–45 minutes. Smash berries. Strain all through a fine mesh strainer and add 1 cup honey, or adjust to taste. Bottle and store in the refrigerator. Will last 2–3 months when refrigerated. ❧

Ginger Echinacea Syrup

This is a truly delicious syrup that's very effective. Other herbs can be added, such as wild cherry bark and licorice for cough, valerian for restlessness, and elecampane for respiratory infection.

> 1 part fresh gingerroot, grated or chopped
> 1 part dried echinacea root

Follow the directions for making syrup on page 29. Ginger is very warming; if the syrup is too "hot" for your child's taste, serve the syrup diluted in warm water or tea. ❧

Feed a Cold?

What and how much a sick child eats will greatly affect the degree of illness. All dairy products, especially milk and ice cream, tend to make the symptoms of a cold worse. Sugar-rich foods should be avoided. So should orange juice, in spite of what the glossy ads say. A large, ice-cold glass of orange juice, no matter how good it tastes, is very acidic and will create more mucus and congestion. Instead, try hot lemonade made with fresh squeezed lemon juice, a pinch of ginger, and a little honey or maple syrup to sweeten. Lemons provide vitamin C, are alkalizing, and will help prevent illness.

Grandma's chicken soup (or, if you're a vegetarian, miso or vegetable broth) is really the best thing to eat when you have a cold or flu. The mineral-rich broth, the fluid, and the warmth are all beneficial. I often add medicinal herbs directly to the soup base. Astragalus, dandelion root, burdock root, echinacea, and even prince ginseng, can be added for extra strength, nourishment, and vitality.

Treating a Runny Nose and Head Congestion

A favorite "instant" remedy for sinus congestion and runny noses is an old-time herbal steam. Heat a large pot of water until steaming, add a drop or two of eucalyptus oil, and have the child inhale this steam. Cover the child's head and the pan with a large towel and treat for 5 to 10 minutes or until the sinuses open up. Instruct the child to keep her eyes closed tight, as the herbal oils can make them water and cause some discomfort. Because you're using a large container of hot water, always stay by the child while she breathes the herbal steam and be sure young hands don't touch the hot pot (or pour water into a heat-resistant bowl first before adding oils). Do not use the steam for children under 4 years old.

Treating Lung and Chest Congestion

A hot-water bottle placed over the back between the shoulder blades helps loosen up phlegm and deep-seated congestion in the chest. I use an old-fashioned hot-water bottle wrapped in cotton flannel to keep in the heat. It's even more effective if you rub Bag Balm, Vicks VapoRub, or a homemade vapor-type salve over the back and chest. Because the oils can be irritating to the eyes, don't ever let the child rub these salves on himself. Do it yourself — and be careful not to put too much on that tender young skin.

Tea & Tincture for Lung & Chest Congestion

This formula can be made into a tea, syrup, or tincture and is very effective in clearing up bronchial congestion. If making a tea, adjust flavors by adding more licorice, cinnamon, and ginger to the formula. If your child is prone to respiratory infections, make the formula up ahead of time as a tincture.

> 2 parts licorice root
> 1 part echinacea
> 1 part elecampane
> 1 part cinnamon
> ¼ part ginger

Combine ingredients and store in airtight container. To make tea, see directions on page 27. To make tincture, see page 32 for instructions. See chart on page 25 for dosage. 🌿

Insect Bites, Burns, Cuts, and Scratches

Invariably, all children get bee stings, insect bites, cuts, and scratches. These are perfect opportunities to teach them the art of self-care and make them little "healers." Include your children when you're making herbal salves and homemade remedies. Most children love to participate in these activities and are much keener to use a medicine they've made themselves. What's even more fun is to go out with them to pick the common garden "weeds" that are powerful healing plants: plantain, dandelion, burdock, and other of nature's great gifts.

THE VERSATILE ALOE VERA PLANT

This "living pharmacy" is good for burns, cuts, wounds, and rashes. The long, succulent green leaves of this hardy houseplant exude a mucilaginous, soothing gel that is highly regarded as a household remedy. *Note:* Never use aloe vera gel on a staph infection. It will seal in the bacteria, creating a perfect petri-environment for the staph to multiply.

Healing Clay

Clay is composed of mineral-rich deposits accumulated over millions of years. Green clay is particularly rich in minerals and is the one I prefer. You can buy green clay in most natural foods or herb stores, and it is a wonderful healing agent when used alone or in combination with herbs for cuts, wounds, and insect bites. If you happen to have a rich deposit of clay in your area, you might wish to get it analyzed for its mineral content.

    4 parts clay
    1 part organically grown goldenseal powder or
        chaparral powder
    1 part comfrey root powder
    1 part dry aloe vera powder

Mix dry powdered clay with finely powdered herbs. Store in a glass jar. To use, mix a small amount with water to form a paste and apply directly to cuts, wounds, and insect bites.

Alternatively, you can premix the clay and herbal powders into a paste with water. Add a few drops of lavender and tea tree essential oils and store in a glass jar with a tight-fitting lid. If the clay dries out, just remoisten with water.

Treating Burns

The salve recipe on page 68 is the best salve recipe known for first- and even second-degree burns. I'm not even sure where the recipe originated, but it's been circulating for as long as I've been practicing herbalism. It's a must in every household with small children.

Another remedy that I have used on second-degree burns is a mixture of 1 tablespoon honey with 1 or 2 drops peppermint oil. Honey has been used for centuries as an antiseptic dressing for burns. The addition of the peppermint oil helps "cool" the burn. On a minor burn, it will relieve pain almost instantly. The honey also keeps the burn clean and free from infection.

The fresh gel from the aloe vera is easily extracted. Choose a large succulent leaf and slice it carefully off the mother plant. The plant will ooze a gel-like substance and heal itself where you've cut it. Slice along the edge of the leaf lengthwise (cutting only as far as you need to for one application of gel). Scoop out the gel, scraping the skin clean. This gel can be applied directly to any burn, wound, or rash. If you don't use the entire leaf, wrap the remainder in plastic wrap and store it in the refrigerator. It will keep for several months.

Promoting Good Health

Included here are some of my favorite tea recipes for promoting good health in children. Each of the teas tastes delicious and can be drunk either by itself or mixed with fruit juice to sweeten. If there is a particular tea recipe your child most enjoys or needs, I suggest mixing up a quart of the blend to keep on hand. Stored in the refrigerator, it will last several days. In the warmer months keep a bottle of iced herbal tea in the refrigerator.

High C Tea

A wonderfully refreshing blend, High C Tea provides bioflavonoids and vitamin C in an organic, naturally biochelated base so that all the nutrients are readily available for absorption. High levels of vitamins supplied in therapeutic dosages, such as commercial vitamins, may be useful to combat illness, but for daily maintenance a more naturally occurring dose is better for your child.

1 part cinnamon chips	⅛ part orange peel
2 parts lemongrass	1 part spearmint
3 parts hibiscus	a pinch of stevia
4 parts rose hips	

Combine all ingredients and store in an airtight container. Make a tea following the instructions on page 27. This is a tonic, so your child can drink as much of it as wanted.

Calming and Relaxing Tea

This blend is especially useful for calming a fussy child. It is gently soothing and can be used over an extended period of time as a tonic for the nervous system. This blend is also helpful during stressful situations such as colic, fevers, and teething.

2 parts oatstraw
1 part catnip
1 part rose petals
2 parts chamomile
2 parts lemon balm

½ part St.-John's-wort
a pinch of stevia per
   cup of dried herb mix
   (optional)

Combine all ingredients and store in an airtight container. Make a tea following the instructions on page 27. This tonic blend can be safely consumed as often as desired by your child. ✑

Respiratory Tonic Tea

This blend is an effective and tasty tea for building strong, healthy lungs. It is especially helpful for children who have reccurring respiratory problems such as colds, flu, hay fever, asthma, ear infections, and general congestion. This tea is not necessarily the blend you might choose to use in the acute stages of a respiratory infection but, used over a period of time, it will aid in creating a healthy respiratory system.

1 part red clover
   flowers
1 part mullein
1 part coltsfoot

2 parts lemongrass
4 parts rose hips
4 parts fennel
1 part calendula

Combine all ingredients and store in an airtight container. Make a tea following the instructions on page 27. ✑

Cough Be Gone & Sore Throat Syrup

2 parts slippery elm bark

2 parts valerian

2 parts wild cherry bark

2 parts licorice root

4 parts fennel seeds

1 part cinnamon bark

½ part gingerroot

⅛ part orange peel

Combine all ingredients and store in an airtight container. Make a decoction following the instructions on page 27. When finished, prepare syrup as instructed on page 29. See chart on page 25 for dosage.

Recipes for Baby Care Products

Though there is a wonderful variety of natural baby care products on the market these days, it's delightful, simple, and far less costly to make your own.

When I first started making my own baby products I was a young, single, working mom. Cost was certainly a factor to me, but not nearly as important as the purity of the product. The only baby products available were the typical commercial ones, and they were far from natural. So I

THE EARTH MADE GREEN AGAIN

I have a vision of the Earth made green again through the efforts of children. I can see children of all nations planting trees and holding hands around the globe in celebration of the Earth as their home and all children, all people as their family.

— *Richard St. Barbe Baker*

decided to make my own. Thirty years later, these products are still popular and have been used by hundreds of parents and their children. All are 100 percent natural and are easy and fun to make.

Baby's Sweet Sleep Pillow

Create a very special pillow to soothe your infant into a calm, peaceful sleep. These herb pillows have proven helpful for children who have trouble sleeping deeply and restfully and who are disturbed by troubling dreams. Use soft, natural fabric for your pillow covering; flannel is wonderful!

    1 part chamomile
    1 part lavender
    1 part roses
    1 part hops
    1–2 drops lavender essential oil

Combine the herbs in a bowl. Add a drop or two of lavender essential oil and mix well. Stitch three sides of a 6 by 6-inch cotton "pillow," leaving one end open for stuffing. Fill abundantly with the herbal sleep mixture. Place near baby's head to help promote peaceful, aromatic sleep. ✺

Baby's Bath Herbs

Use the following mixture in the bathwater. These herbs are soothing and relaxing — for Mom and Dad, too.

    1 part roses
    2 parts chamomile
    2 parts calendula
    1 part lavender
    2 parts comfrey leaf

Mix all herbs. Place a small handful of the mixture in a cotton bag. Add bag to baby's bath, allowing the herbs to steep in the water. Use the fragrant herbal bag as a washcloth. ✺

Bottoms Up Salve

This is my very favorite salve recipe for diaper rash, cuts and scrapes, and irritated skin. If you don't have the time to steep for two weeks or if there's not much sun, let the herbs steep in the olive oil in a double boiler over very low heat for several hours. Check frequently to be sure the oil is not over-heating and burning the herbs.

    1 part comfrey leaf
    1 part comfrey root
    1 part St.-John's-wort flower
    1 part calendula flower
    olive oil
    grated beeswax

1. Combine herbs and store in an airtight container. Make a solar infusion by steeping 2 ounces of the herb mixture in 1 pint of olive oil for 2 weeks. (See page 28 for instructions on making a solar infusion.) This will create about 2 cups of herbal oil.

2. At the end of 2 weeks, place mixture in a double boiler and warm for 1 hour over *very* low heat. Strain.

3. To each cup of warm herbal oil, add ¼ cup of grated beeswax. You might need to warm the oil a little longer to melt the beeswax.

4. When the beeswax is melted, check for desired consistency; place 1 tablespoon of the mixture in the refrigerator for a few minutes. If the salve is too hard, add little more oil; if too soft, add a little more beeswax. Pour into a glass jar. The salve does not need to be refrigerated and will last for months (or years) if stored in a cool area.

Baby Powder

This is an excellent daily baby powder. You may wish to lightly scent the powder, but use only pure essential oil and be certain it is nonirritating to the child's sensitive skin. Orange oil is light and refreshing and often used as the scent for baby powders.

  2 parts white clay (available in natural foods stores and ceramic supply stores)
  2 parts arrowroot powder
  ¼ part slippery elm or marsh mallow root powder
  ¼ part comfrey root powder

1. Mix the ingredients together and place in a shaker bottle, such as a spice jar.

2. To treat diaper rash, add to this mixture ⅛ part organically grown goldenseal powder, ⅛ part myrrh powder, and ⅛ part echinacea. Apply as a powder, or mix into a thin paste and apply as a poultice to the rash. 🦋

Baby Oil

This is excellent all-purpose oil and is wonderful to rub on baby after baths. It also makes a great massage oil for babies.

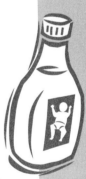

  1 pint apricot or almond oil
  ½ ounce roses
  1 ounce chamomile
  ½ ounce comfrey leaf

1. Mix herbs and oil together and let sit in a glass jar with tight-fitting lid for 2 weeks in a warm, sunny spot.

2. For a stronger oil, pour into the top of a double boiler. Slowly warm the mixture over very low heat for 1 hour. Strain and bottle. You may lightly scent with a few drops of pure essential oil such as lavender, rose, or chamomile. Use at room temperature only. Store in a cool place. 🦋

Recommended Reading

Bove, Dr. Mary. *An Encyclopedia of Natural Healing for Children and Infants.* New Canaan, CT: Keats Publishing, 1996.

de Bairacli Levy, Juliette. *Nature's Children.* Woodstock, NY: Ash Tree Publishing, 1997.

Dodt, Colleen. *Natural BabyCare.* Pownal, VT: Storey Communications, 1997.

Gardner, Joy. *The New Healing Yourself: Natural Remedies for Adults and Children.* Freedom, CA: Crossing Press, 1989.

Mazzarella, Barbara. *Bach Flower Remedies for Children.* Rochester, VT: Healing Arts Press, 1994.

McIntyre, Anne. *The Herbal for Mother and Child.* Rockport, MA: Element Press, 1992.

Romm, Aviva Jill. *Natural Healing for Babies and Children.* Freedom, CA: Crossing Press, 1996.

Theiss, Barbara, and Peter Theiss. *The Family Herbal.* Rochester, VT: Healing Arts Press, 1989.

White, Linda and Sunny Mavor. *Kids, Herbs, Health.* Loveland, CO: Interweave Press, 1999.

Zand, Janet, Rachel Walton, and Robert Roundtree. *Smart Medicine for a Healthier Child.* Garden City Park, NY: Avery Publishing Group, 1994.

Resources

Herbs

Frontier Herbs
P.O. Box 299
Norway, IA 52318
(800) 669-3275
Frontier is a wholesale supplier, but offers price breaks for individual buyers. Inquire.

Green Mountain Herbs
PO Box 532
Putney, VT 05436
(888) 4GRNMTS

Healing Spirits
9198 State Route 415
Avoca, NY 14809
(607) 566-2701
One of the best sources of ethically wildcrafted and organically grown herbs.

Jean's Greens
119 Sulphur Springs Road
Newport, NY 13146
(315) 845-6500
A wonderful selection of fresh and dried organic and wildcrafted herbs. Also, materials needed for making herbal products.

Mountain Rose
20818 High Street
North San Juan, CA 95960
(800) 879-3337
Mountain Rose supplies bulk herbs, beeswax, books, oils, and containers.

Trinity Herbs
P.O. Box 1001
Graton, CA 95444
(707) 824-2040
Trinity is a small wholesale herb company that sells bulk herbs in quantities of one pound or more.

Wild Weeds
1302 Camp Weott Road
Ferndale, CA 95536
(800) 553-9453
A small herbal emporium.

Woodland Essences
PO Box 206
Cold Brook, NY 13324
(315) 845-1515

Handmade Herbal Products

Avena Botanicals
20 Mill Street
Rockland, ME 04841

Equinox Botanicals
33446 McCumber Road
Rutland, OH 45775

Green Terrestrial
P.O. Box 266
Milton, NY 12547

Herb Pharm
Box 116
Williams, OR 97544

Herbalists and Alchemists
P.O. Box 553
Broadway, NJ 08808

Sage Mountain Herb Products
General Delivery
Lake Elmore, VT 05657
(802) 888-7278
Rosemary Gladstar's company.

Simpler's Botanicals
P.O. Box 39
Forestville, CA 95436

Zand Herbal Products
Products available in most natural foods and herb stores across the country.

Educational Resources

The California School of Herbal Studies
P.O. Box 39
Forestville, CA 95476
One of the oldest and most respected herb schools in the United States, founded by Rosemary Gladstar in 1982.

Herb Research Foundation
1007 Pearl Street, Suite 200
Boulder, CO 80302

Rocky Mountain Center for Botanical Studies
1705 Fourteenth Street, #287
Boulder, CO 80302
Offers excellent programs for beginners, as well as advanced clinical training programs.

Sage Mountain Retreat Center and Botanical Sanctuary
P.O. Box 420
East Barre, VT 05649
Apprentice programs and classes with Rosemary Gladstar and other well-known herbalists.

The Science and Art of Herbalism: A Home Study Course
by Rosemary Gladstar
P.O. Box 420
East Barre, VT 05649
An in-depth study of herbs, emphasizing the foundations of herbalism, wildcrafting, Earth awareness, and herbal preparation and formulation.

For a small fee, the following organizations can provide information on classes, seminars, and correspondnce courses offered throughout the United States.

American Herbalist Guild (AHG)
Box 746555
Arvada, CO 80006

American Herb Association (AHA)
P.O. Box 1673
Nevada City, CA 95959

The Northeast Herb Association
P.O. Box 10
Newport, NY 13416

Herb Newsletters

The American Herb Association Newsletter
P.O. Box 1673
Nevada City, CA 95959

Business of Herbs
North Winds Farm
439 Pondersona Way
Jemez Springs, NM 87025

Foster's Botanical and Herb Reviews
P.O. Box 106
Eureka Springs, AR 72632

HerbalGram
P.O. Box 201660
Austin, TX 78720

The Herb Quarterly
P.O. Box 548
Boiling Springs, PA 17007

Herbs for Health and *The Herb Companion*
201 East Fourth Street
Loveland, CO 80537

Medical Herbalism
P.O. Box 33080
Portland, OR 97233

Planetary Formula Newsletter
c/o Roy Upton
P.O. Box 533
Soquel, CA 95073

United Plant Savers
P.O. Box 420
East Barre, VT 05649

Wild Foods Forum
4 Carlisle Way NE
Atlanta, GA 30308

United Plant Savers At-Risk List

United Plant Savers (UpS) is a nonprofit, grassroots organization dedicated to preserving native American medicinal plants and the land that they grow on. An organization for herbalists and people who love and use plants, our purpose is to ensure the future of our rich diversity of medicinal plants through organic cultivation, sustainable wildcrafting practices, creating botanical sanctuaries for medicinal plant conservation, and reestablishing native plant communities in their natural environments.

The following herbs have been designated as "UpS At Risk" due to overharvesting, loss of habitat, or by nature of their innate rareness or sensitivity. UpS is not asking for a moratorium on the use of these herbs, but rather is asking for a concerted effort by all those who use plants as medicine to seek sustainable alternatives; that is, grow your own, buy from reputable companies, or substitute other herbs whenever possible.

American Ginseng (*Panax quinquefolius*)

Black Cohosh (*Cimicifuga racemosa*)

Bloodroot (*Sanguinaria canadensis*)

Blue Cohosh (*Caulophyllum thalictroides*)

Echinacea (*Echinacea* species)

Goldenseal (*Hydrastis canadensis*)

Helonias Root (*Chamaelirium luteum*)

Kava Kava (*Piper methysticum*) (Hawaii only)

Lady's-Slipper (*Cypripedium* species)

Lomatium (*Lomatium dissectum*)

Osha (*Ligusticum porteri* and related species)

Partridgeberry (*Mitchella repens*)

Peyote (*Lophophora williamsii*)

Slippery elm (*Ulmus rubra*)

Sundew (*Drosera* species)

Trillium, Beth root (*Trillium* species)

True Unicorn (*Aletris farinosa*)

Venus's-flytrap (*Dionaea muscipula*)

Wild Yam (*Dioscorea villosa* and related species)

For more information on United Plant Savers and how you can become involved in "Planting the Future," contact United Plant Savers, P.O. Box 98, East Barre, VT 05649; (802) 479-9825; E-mail: info@www.plantsavers.org.

Index

Other Storey Books
You Will Enjoy

Also in th Rosemary Gladstar's series: *Herbal Remedies for Men's Health,* ISBN 1-58017-151-6; *Herbs for Longevity and Well-Being,* ISBN 1-58017-154-0; *Herbs for Natural Beauty,* ISBN 1-58017-152-4; *Herbs for Reducing Stress and Anxiety,* ISBN 1-58017-155-9; and *Herbs for the Home Medicine Chest,* ISBN 1-58017-156-7.

Healing with Herbs, by Penelope Ody. This visual introduction to the world of herbal medicine offers clear, illustrated instructions for growing, preparing, and administering healing herbs to relieve a variety of ailments. 160 pages. Hardcover. ISBN 1-58017-144-3.

The Herbal Home Remedy Book, by Joyce A. Wardwell. Readers will discover how to use 25 common herbs to make simple herbal remedies. Native American legends and folklore are spread throughout the book. 176 pages. Paperback. ISBN 1-58017-016-1.

Herbal Remedy Gardens, by Dorie Byers. An introduction to more than 20 herbs, their medicinal uses, and propagation and harvesting techniques, this book includes dozens of easy-to-make recipes for common ailments. Thirty-eight illustrated garden plans offer choices for customizing a garden to fit your special health needs. 224 pages. Paperback. ISBN 1-58017-095-1.

Natural BabyCare, by Colleen K. Dodt. Learn special tips and try your hand at simple recipes for products made to soothe and care for your baby. 144 pages. Paperback. ISBN 0-88266-953-2.

Natural First Aid, by Brigitte Mars. This book offers natural first aid suggestions for everything from ant bites to wounds. Readers will also find recipes for simple home remedies using herbs, vitamins, essential oils, and foods. Includes an herb profile section detailing the healing properties of common herbs. 128 pages. Paperback. ISBN 1-58017-147-8.

These and other Storey Books are available at your bookstore, farm store, garden center, or directly from Storey Books, Schoolhouse Road, Pownal, Vermont 05261, or by calling 1-800-441-5700. Or visit our Web site at www.storey.com.